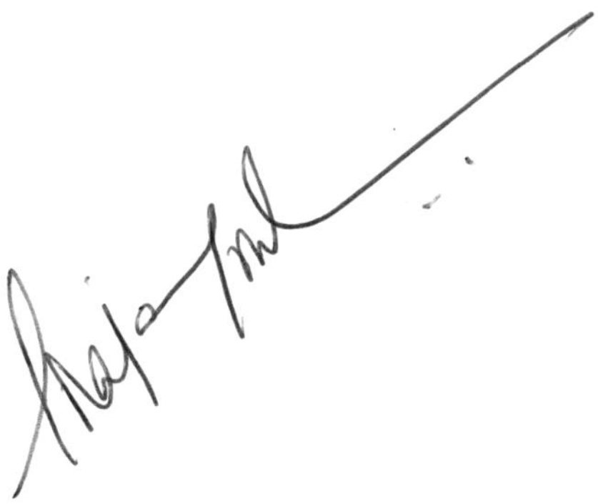

Understanding the Biology of Mental Disorders

Understanding the Biology of Mental Disorders

Timothy G. Dinan

Department of Psychological Medicine
St Bartholomew's and
The Royal London School of Medicine
London, UK

SCIENCE PRESS

Published by Science Press Limited, 34–42 Cleveland Street, London, W1P 6LB, UK

British Library Cataloguing in Publication Data.

A catalogue record for this book is available from the British Library.

ISBN 1-85873-165-8

PZ796

This book represents the findings of its authors and is not necessarily the opinion of Lilly Psychiatry — a subsidiary of Eli Lilly & Company.

Although every effort has been made to ensure that drug doses and other information are presented accurately in this publication, the ultimate responsibility rests with the prescribing physician. Neither the publishers nor the authors can be held responsible for errors or for any consequences arising from the use of the information contained herein. Any product mentioned in this publication should be used in accordance with the prescribing information prepared by the manufacturers. No claims or endorsements are made for any drug or compound under clinical investigation.

Project editor: Hannah Moss
Illustrations: Resolution Design Ltd and Matthew McCutcheon
Typesetter: Paul Angliss
Cover designer: Claire Huntley
Production: Kate Oldfield
Printed in Spain

10 9 8 7 6 5 4 3 2 1

Contents

Contributors

Timothy G. Dinan
Lucinda Scott
Frances E. Burnett
Jogin H. Thakore
Department of Psychological Medicine
St Bartholomew's Hospital
London, UK

Michael Gill
Department of Old Age Psychiatry
Brian A. Lawlor
Department of Psychiatry
Trinity Centre for Health Sciences
St. James' Hospital
Dublin, Ireland

Lyn Pilowsky
Michael Travis
Kathryn Abel
James V. Lucey
Department of Psychological Medicine
Institute of Psychiatry
London, UK

Nicholas J. Coupland
Department of Psychiatry
University of Alberta
Edmonton, Alberta, Canada

David J. Nutt
University of Bristol Psychopharmacology Unit
School of Medical Sciences
Bristol, UK

Hanno Pijl
A. Edo Meinders
Department of General Internal Medicine
Leiden University Hospital
Leiden, The Netherlands

Michael Kirby
Department of Old Age Psychiatry
St Vincent's Hospital
Dublin, Ireland

Preface

Over the past decade, psychiatry has seen a greater emphasis on biological processes and is once again entering mainstream medicine. This shift towards a biological perspective is shown in the examinations of the Royal College of Psychiatrists, the increasing strength of organizations such as the American College of Neuropsychopharmacology and the appointment of several neurobiologists to senior chairs, which were formerly occupied by social psychiatrists. While welcoming this altered perception, the important role of both a social and psychological perspective in clinical management should not be diminished. This book provides a concise overview of biological psychiatry for trainee psychiatrists and senior colleagues who wish to update themselves with these recent advances.

Pharmacological progress has always been at the heart of biological psychiatry. The development of chlorpromazine in the early 1950s marks the greatest watershed in somatic psychiatry. That the drug was an effective antipsychotic agent was shown soon after its synthesis, and before long it was available throughout Europe and North America. The late 1950s saw the development of haloperidol and in the 1960s numerous other antipsychotic agents were synthesized. Nonetheless, none of these events surpassed the original discovery of chlorpromazine. Similar fortuitous advances took place in the 1950s with the recognition that monoamine oxidase inhibitors had antidepressant effects and that the initial tricyclic compounds also possessed antidepressant properties. From the 1950s until relatively recently, progress in our understanding of biological processes, and pharmacological interventions has been rather slow. The development of the selective serotonin reuptake inhibitors and their launch in the 1980s marked another milestone, as did the recognition that the antipsychotic agent clozapine had a broader spectrum of therapeutic action than traditional neuroleptic drugs. Several new atypical antipsychotic agents, pharmacologically modelled on clozapine, are now available. Their presence is a major advance in the management of schizophrenia.

Our understanding of biological processes relating to psychiatric illness has never kept apace with pharmacological advances. Nonetheless, there are significant grounds for optimism at present. With molecular biology techniques it is now becoming possible to determine the gene defects underlying some of the most debilitating mental illnesses. This book provides the reader with the basic terminology used in molecular genetics and provides an insight into future possibilities. Neuroimaging has come a long way since the development of the initial computed tomography scanners. We are now in an era of functional imaging with the development of functional magnetic resonance imaging, positron emission tomography and single photon emission tomography. These technologies are advancing at a rapid pace, and offer a breath-taking capacity to study the human brain at a physiological level, without invasive procedures. The abundant literature emanating from this area is a testament to the volume of research being conducted.

With major neurochemical advances, the complex neurotransmitter pathways in the human brain and the second messenger processes lying behind receptor systems are now better understood. Future generations of drugs will probably target second messenger systems rather than the surface receptors. Neuroendocrinology has also shown significant progress. Neuroendocrinologists have gained a greater insight into the biological processes underlying the stress response. Clearly most psychiatric illnesses either occur in a setting of stress or are exacerbated by stress. Therefore a greater understanding of stress biology will have a major influence on the management of psychiatric illness.

This book is not all-embracing but provides a review of the key issues in biological psychiatry. Many readers may find the issues sufficiently stimulating to look at more comprehensive texts or original articles. If this book inspires a few junior colleagues to pursue a career in biological psychiatry it will, I feel, have been a major success.

Timothy G. Dinan

Molecular genetics

Michael Gill

Classic genetic background

Kraepelin distinguished manic depression from dementia praecox (schizophrenia), and described its genetic component or 'heredity taint'. Despite this, early genetic studies included manic depression or bipolar disorder with unipolar depression, treating the affective disorders as a single entity. Leonhard [1] divided affective disorders into two categories for the purposes of his genetic studies: bipolar affective disorder or manic depression, which has manic and depressive episodes, and unipolar disorders, which have only depression. Leonhard found that probands with bipolar disorder had more bipolar disorder among their relatives than did probands with unipolar depression. Perris [2] and Angst [3] confirmed this familial distinction that the relatives tended to have the same disorder as was found in the probands. Furthermore, Perris suggested that hereditary factors are more pronounced in bipolar than in unipolar disorders.

In genetic terms, a phenotype is the observable expression of an underlying genotype, possibly influenced by the environment. In the absence of a biochemical marker of the disease, a definition of the symptoms and signs that make up the phenotype is required. This applies to classic genetic studies, such as the family studies mentioned above, and to twin and adoption studies. It also applies to the molecular genetic work discussed later in this chapter. For a disease with a variable age of onset and a remitting and relapsing course, the phenotype is defined as a lifetime diagnosis. The validity of the clinical diagnosis as a definition of the phenotype remains unknown, but the reliability has improved considerably with the advent of research interviews, such as SCAN (schedules for clinical assessment in neuropsychiatry) and operational diagnoses [4].

In a review of 10 studies performed since 1982 Mitchell *et al.* [5] show a higher risk of affective disorders in relatives of bipolar probands (1.5–14.5%), compared with relatives of control individuals (0.2–1.3%). Weissman *et al.* [6] studied the morbidity risk in families of bipolar I (depressive and manic episodes) and bipolar II (depressive and 'hypomanic' episodes). They found an increased risk of both bipolar I and bipolar II disorders in families of bipolar I probands compared with relatives of control individuals. For relatives of bipolar II probands, however, the studies found a higher risk of bipolar II (9.8% compared with 1.1% control) but no increased risk of bipolar I (0.9% compared with 0.2% control). These results suggest a stronger familial component in bipolar I disorder. Rates of unipolar depression are also increased in the relatives of bipolar I probands (7.8–22%) compared with the relatives of control individuals (4.6–5.9%). Blacker and Tsuang [7] concluded that 65–74% of the unipolar relatives of bipolar probands must be genetically related to the bipolar cases. In contrast, they calculated that only 5% of the UP relatives of controls are 'genetically' bipolar.

For some disorders, age of onset has defined aetiological subtypes. For example, for Alzheimer's disease the risk of morbidity is three times greater in first degree relatives of early onset (<30 years) Alzheimer's probands than relatives of those with late onset (>30 years). Alternatively, early age of onset may be a mark of severity of disease, in the context of a polygenic mode of transmission. The role, if any, of age of onset in defining genetic subtypes in bipolar or unipolar affective disorder is not yet understood.

Twin studies

Using twin registers as a source of data, studies have reported significantly higher concordance in monozygotic than dizygotic twins when one twin had an affective disorder. Bertelsen *et al.* [8] studied the National Psychiatric Twin Register and found the rate of bipolar concordance to be 61% in monozygotic twins and 8% in dizygotic twins. Additional co-twins had unipolar depression, making the concordance rates for affective disorder, starting with a bipolar co-twin, 79% and 19% for monozygotic and dizygotic pairs respectively. In an interesting and important study, Bertelsen and Gottesman [9] studied the frequency of bipolar affective disorder in the offspring of monozygotic twins, of which only one was affected with bipolar disorder. They found that 20.7% of the offspring of the ill twins had affective disorder, but 24.7% of the offspring of the well co-twins also had affective disorder, suggesting the presence of unexpressed genetic factors in the well co-twin, which are passed on to offspring. The rate of affective disorder in the unaffected co-twin is very similar to the 21% found in the offspring of probands with bipolar disorder.

Adoption studies

Mendlewicz and Rainer [10] investigated data on 39 bipolar adoptees, obtained from out-patient and in-patient medical records. The frequencies of psychopathological symptoms in their biological and adoptive parents were compared with each other, and with control parents. First, with parents of patients with BP who were not adopted; second, with biological and adopted parents of healthy adoptees, and finally with parents of individuals who contracted poliomyelitis in childhood. They found significantly more affective disorder among the biological relatives of BP adoptees compared with the adoptive relatives. The rate of AD in the biological relatives of BP adoptees (28%) was similar to that in the relatives of BP nonadoptees (26%), but greater than that among the adoptive relatives (12%) or control individuals.

In summary, family, twin and adoption studies individually and in combination, support the hypothesis of a genetic component in affective disorders, especially in bipolar disorder. Different diagnostic methods and potential ascertainment bias make the accurate calculation of the size of the genetic component difficult.

Modes of transmission

Clearly the rates of illness in relatives of BP probands do not support a Mendelian model of transmission for the disease as a whole. Indeed, only a few families show a pattern of transmission consistent with simple Mendelian inheritance and it is possible that these occur by chance. Ruling out a simple Mendelian model, several more complex models can be considered.

Next to a Mendelian model, the simplest model of transmission is the single major locus (SML). The oligogenic model postulates that a few genes (5–10) act collectively to determine a disease. The polygenic model postulates that the disease is determined by many genes each contributing in a small way. The polygenic model suits quantitative traits, but for a dichotomous disease or normal trait an underlying liability or trait that is not directly measurable is postulated. Only those whose liability exceeds a certain threshold demonstrate the disease. Using this additional facility, the polygenic model can be extended into a multifactorial model where disease is determined by both polygenes and environmental factors. Experience with other diseases such as Alzheimer's disease, however, suggests that pure single major locus, polygenic and multifactorial models are unlikely to exist. Therefore, a mixed model is plausible, possibly in the form of a single major locus operating with a polygenic background [11]. In this model, the penetrance of the major gene is influenced by the action of polygenes or multiple environmental factors.

With the family data presently available it has not been possible to determine a clear mode of transmission. It is doubtful whether it would be possible even with data from a family study considerably larger than any yet published. Further progress in clarifying the mode of transmission will require a different approach.

Update on molecular genetic studies

The availability of DNA technology, and the discovery of highly polymorphic DNA markers have made it possible to locate, identify and characterize genes for almost any genetic disorder that has a simple or Mendelian mode of transmission. Recently, molecular genetic methods have identified genes of major effect in conditions previously thought to be polygenic, such as Alzheimer's disease [12], Hirschsprung's disease [13], and migraine [14]. More importantly, susceptibility genes (see Oligogenic Model above) have also been identified, for example, in Alzheimer's disease [15] and diabetes mellitus [16]. There are two main strategies currently used in searching for susceptibility loci in 'complex genetic diseases' such as bipolar affective disorder. These are genetic linkage studies and genetic association studies

Genetic linkage studies

Linkage studies investigate possible co-segregation of a genetic marker and a disorder, in one or more families. Therefore, linkage studies have two main aims: first, to detect departure from independent assortment, and second, to estimate the amount of recombination between the marker and the putative disease gene. Recombination takes the value 0.5 when the two loci are unlinked, and a value between 0 and 0.5 when there is some evidence of linkage. As a statistical measure of the strength of the apparent co-segregation the Lod score of Morton (Log of the odds ratio) is used [17]. This ratio compares the likelihood that apparent co-segregation is due to linkage, with the likelihood that the apparent co-segregation is due to chance. For Mendelian disorders, a Lod score of 3 or more is the point at which linkage is concluded and a score of –2 or less is the point at which linkage is excluded.

The sib-pair method of studying linkage [18,19] does not depend on the description of the disease locus and is seen as an alternative to the Lod score method in examining complex genetic diseases. Normally, at any given locus, pairs of affected siblings share two, one, or no parental alleles, 25%, 50% and 25% of the time respectively. If a disease susceptibility locus and a genetic marker are linked, the marker alleles are shared more often than expected. In addition to being 'model free', the affected sib-pair method and a modification known as the relative pair methods have several practical advantages: their unit of study is smaller than extended pedigrees, families with clear diagnoses can be selected, and the statistics are easier to analyse than for the Lod score method. In bipolar affective disorders, the absence of strong *a priori* evidence for a single gene and external validity of clinical diagnoses are major difficulties for linkage analysis. In theory, however, either the Lod score or sib-pair method will detect even genes of minor effect, providing there are sufficient families available to study. In the studies below, the term exclusion is taken to mean 'exclusion under the model and assumptions of the study'.

Genetic association studies

Studies of genetic association may also be used to detect susceptibility genes in complex genetic disorders. Unlike linkage studies, which test for co-segregation within a family, these studies test for association between particular alleles of a polymorphism and the disease phenotype. Therefore, association studies require a large sample of unrelated, affected individuals and controls. If a mutation contributes to a disease, it will occur more frequently in patients than controls. Alleles adjacent to the mutation will also occur more frequently in patients. This is because recombination occurs infrequently within a short distance on a chromosome, thus preserving the association between the mutation and particular alleles of closely related polymorphisms over many generations. This phenomenon is known as linkage disequilibrium [20]. Whether two polymorphisms are in linkage disequilibrium or not depends on the distance between them, the frequency of recombination in the region, and the number of generations since their co-occurrence on the same strand of DNA.

Genetic association is only likely to be detected in markers that are close to, or that are part of, the mutation, and therefore association studies are currently confined to investigating markers within or close to genes. This is in contrast to linkage studies, which may systematically search the whole genome. It should also be noted that no clear candidate genes for bipolar affective disorder exist and approximately 50 000 genes are expressed preferentially or exclusively in the brain.

Gene-finding strategies

Currently three molecular genetic approaches are used to find genes. The first is to study 'candidate' genes, using both linkage analysis in pedigrees and association analysis in unrelated affected individuals and controls. This is also known as functional cloning. The second approach is linkage analysis within regions of the genome suggested by a suspected mode of transmission, a cytogenetic abnormality, or the preliminary results of a genome scan. The third strategy, requiring large resources, is a systematic genome search to detect genes of major effect using parametric or non-parametric analyses (Fig. 1.1). The latter strategies are also known as positional cloning.

Chromosome 11

The short arm of chromosome 11 generated much interest following the publication of a study by Egeland *et al.* [40]. This finding arose from a random search strategy (see page 6). However, the tyrosine hydroxylase (TH) gene is located within the region studied by Egeland's group. TH is a limiting enzyme in the synthesis of monoamines and, as such, is a plausible candidate gene for affective disorders. Leboyer *et al.* [20] reported an association between BP and polymorphisms flanking the TH locus, using a sample of 50 patients and control individuals. Todd

Candidate genes and regions, summary of linkage and association studies

Gene	Region	Study	Linkage	Association
DRD1	5q	Mitchell *et al.*, 1992 [21]		–
DRD2	11q	Byerley *et al.*, 1990 [22]	–	
		Mitchell *et al.*, 1992 [21]	–	
DRD3	3q	Mitchell et al., 1993 [23]	–	
		Shaikh *et al.*, 1993 [24]		–
DRD4	11p	Nanko *et al.*, 1994 [25]	+	
		Lim *et al.*, 1994 [26]		–
DRD5	4p	Sherrington *et al.*, 1993 [27]	–	
DRD5	4p	Byerley *et al.*, 1994 [28]	–	
DRD2 DRD4,TH	11q 11p	De Bruyn *et al.*, 1994 [29]	–	
DRD4,TH	11p	Lim *et al.*, 1993 [30]	+	
		Sidenberg *et al.*, 1994 [31]	+	
MAOA,MAOB	Xp	Lim *et al.*, 1994 [32]		+
DBH	9q3.4	Ewald *et al.*, 1994 [33]	–	
TH	11p	Todd & O'Malley, 1989 [34]		–
		Nothen *et al.*, 1990 [35]		–
		Leboyer *et al.*, 1990 [20]		+
		Gill *et al.*, 1991 [36]		–
		Korner *et al.*, 1994 [37]		–
		Byerley *et al.*, 1992 [38]	+	
Darier's locus	12q	Dawson *et al.*, 1994 [39]	+	

Fig. 1.1 *Candidate genes and regions, summary of linkage and association studies. + indicates some degree of positive findings but not necessarily significant. – indicates negative findings.*

and O'Malley [34] had already reported the frequency of alleles from the two polymorphisms in a sample of 18 patients and 27 controls and found no differences. Similarly Korner *et al.* [41], Nothen *et al.* [35] and Gill *et al.* [36] failed to show a significant association in larger samples. A combined study from the British and German groups also failed to find any evidence of the putative association [37].

In linkage studies of TH polymorphisms Byerley *et al.* [38] could not exclude linkage between BP and TH in one of their eight pedigrees reporting a Lod score of 0.79, recombination = 0 at TH and 1.07 at the insulin locus. Similarly, Lim *et al.* [30] found small positive Lod scores at TH and the nearby dopamine D4 receptor (DRD4) in two out of six large families. Sidenberg *et al.* [31] reported an analysis of the Old Order Amish family and chromosome 11p polymorphisms. The candidate genes for TH and the dopamine D4 receptor gene (DRD4), located at 11p15.5 region, showed small positive Lod scores 0.63 at recombination = 0.10 for TH. Absence of linkage between TH, INS, HRAS markers and manic depression in a Belgian pedigree was reported by Mendlewicz *et al.* [42].

De Bruyn *et al.* [29] reported non-linkage of bipolar illness to TH, tyrosinase, D2 and D4 receptor gene polymorphisms on chromosome 11. The study used both Lod score (parametric) and affected sib-pair (nonparametric) methods of investigation.

Dopamine receptor genes

Many molecular genetic studies in Alzheimer's disease have used polymorphic markers within or near the five dopamine receptor genes. Even though these genes have a potential pathogenic role, all studies have been negative. Linkage analyses of the D1, D2, D3 dopamine receptor genes have been consistently negative [21–23,43]. Association studies of the same receptor genes have also shown no evidence of allelic association [24,44]. Two research groups reported a lack of association between dopamine D4 receptor variants and BP disorders [26,45]. Sherrington *et al.* [27] found no linkage between bipolar and the D5 dopamine receptor gene in five Icelandic pedigrees. Their analysis showed a strongly negative Lod score in three of the pedigrees. Similarly, Byerley *et al.* [28] showed no evidence of linkage to D5 markers. Linkage studies have been carried out between affective disorder and polymorphisms of dopamine DRD2,

DRD3 and DRD4 receptor genes in four Japanese pedigrees [25]. Linkages of DRD2 and DRD3 have been excluded, but the authors could not exclude linkage to DRD4.

Candidate regions

Dawson *et al.* [39] investigated the region on chromosome 12 found previously to be linked to the Darier's locus [46]. The same authors [47] had reported a pedigree in which five members had both Darier's disease and affective disorder. The linkage data reported by Dawson *et al.* [39] was inconclusive but not entirely negative.

X chromosome

In the past 30 years there have been many reports of apparent co-segregation of BP disorders with polymorphic markers in the X chromosome [48–50]. However, several studies did not find any suggestion of linkage to Xq27 and Xq28 markers in their pedigrees [51,52]. Linkage of an AD locus with CB and G6PD would be consistent as both marker loci lie close together in the Xq28 region (Fig. 1.2).

Using a marker at the coagulation factor 9 (F9) locus, Mendlewicz *et al.* [54] reported possible linkage between this locus (Xq27) and AD in 11 pedigrees. The maximum Lod score was 3.1 at recombination = 0.11. They suggested that a BP locus might be linked to CB and loosely linked to factor 9. Supporting this hypothesis, Gill *et al.* [55] reported cosegregation of bipolar disorders and Christmas disease (factor 9 deficiency) in a UK pedigree. Additionally, Lucotte *et al.* [56] found evidence for linkage between BP and factor 9 in a single, large, French pedigree (Lod score = 3.91, recombination = 0).

Appearing perhaps to finally confirm previous reports of X-linkage, Baron *et al.* [53] used colour blindness and G6PD markers in five Jewish pedigrees and reported Lod scores of 7.52 assuming homogeneity, and 9.17 assuming heterogeneity. This was not, however, as many hoped, the end of the linkage detection phase, as the same group [57] re-examined X-linked inheritance of affective disorders in three of these Israeli pedigrees and reported greatly diminished support for linkage of BP disorders to more highly polymorphic DNA markers in the G6PD region.

Both monoamine oxidase (MAO)-A and MAO-B genes have been mapped to Xp11.12–Xp11.4 and are closely linked. Lim *et al.* [32] reported the results of an association study in 59 unrelated bipolar patients and their matched controls. They found a weak, but significant, genetic association between manic depression and MAO-A gene polymorphisms.

Apart from evidence of apparent co-segregation, little support is provided from the published pedigrees for the X-linked mode of inheritance for BP [58]. Hebebrand concluded that formal genetic criteria for an X-linked dominant mode of inheritance are absent in BP disorder, and that the existing X-linkage studies do not provide sufficient evidence to overcome this absence. He suggested that the normally accepted criteria to conclude linkage in a Lod score study of disorders with an uncertain mode of inheritance need to be addressed.

Chromosome 18

Interest in chromosome 18 began when, during the course of a genome scan using 22 bipolar families, Berrettini *et al.* [59] reported excess sharing of alleles among affected sibling pairs. Lod scores were not significant under either dominant or recessive models. This led the authors to speculate that mutations at the same gene might, in different families, segregate as either dominant or recessive.

X-chromosome linkage studies

Marker	Region	Reference	Linkage
CB,G6PD	Xq28	Baron *et al.*, 1987 [53]	+
CB,F9	Xq27	Mendlewicz *et al.*, 1987 [54]	+
		Gershon *et al.*, 1979 [51]	–
		Gejman *et al.*, 1990 [52]	–
F9	Xq27	Gill *et al.*, 1992 [55]	+
		Lucotte *et al.*, 1992 [56]	+
CB,F9	Xq27	Baron *et al.*, 1993 [57]	+
CB		Mendlewicz *et al.*, 1972 [48]	+
		Mendlewicz & Fleiss, 1974 [49]	+
G6PD,CB	Xq27-28	Mendlewicz *et al.*, 1980 [50]	+

Fig. 1.2 *X-chromosome linkage studies. + indicates some degree of positive findings but not necessarily significant. – indicates negative findings.*

Individual pedigree Lod scores, maximized for the genetic model, ranged from 1.08 to 2.38. They pointed out two candidate genes, a corticotropin receptor and the alpha subunit of a GTP binding protein, which were localized to this region. Other studies have had mixed success in attempting replication [60] and some have been quite negative [61]. The strongest evidence in support comes from the study by Freimer *et al.* [62] of two large Costa Rican bipolar pedigrees. The Lod scores in the combined pedigrees were greater than 1.6 but less than 3. In a combined analysis of linkage and association, markers D18S554 and D18S70 gave Lod scores of 3.7 and 4.06, respectively. As with the Berrettini study, the area of suggestive Lod scores is very large indeed, stretching over 40 centimorgans, or approximately 40 million basepairs.

Chromosome 4p

Recently, again as a result of a genome scan, Blackwood *et al.* [63] have reported a two point Lod score of 4.1 between the bipolar disorder phenotype and alleles of marker D4S394 in a single multiply affected pedigree, under a dominant mode of inheritance. This finding is strongly significant and suggests that major genes are sufficient to cause the disease in some highly unusual multiply affected pedigrees. Analysis of other large pedigrees is awaited.

Genome searches

The finding of Egeland *et al.* [40], although later withdrawn, was part of a genome search using a single large multiply affected pedigree [64]. This linkage, however, could not be confirmed in American bipolar pedigrees of non Amish origin [65] and in other pedigrees [66,67]. Allowing for the cautious correction suggested by Watt and Edwards [68] to account for the use of many markers, the Lod score was still >3 ($4.32-1.3=3.02$). However, when Egeland's group extended the pedigree and followed it up over a 2 year period, two previously well individuals were now diagnosed as affected. This reduced the Lod score for H-ras from the original 4.32 at recombination $=0$ to 2.46 at recombination $=0.05$. The lateral extension of the pedigree was clearly not linked, and assuming homogeneity within the pedigree as a whole, the total Lod score became negative [69]. Since this episode, and up until recently, few systematic searches have been made.

In a study of classic markers, Ewald *et al.* [33] reported non-linkage between manic depression and 35 classic markers. They found no evidence of linkage with the markers on chromosomes 4q, 9q and 19 for a broad phenotypic model. Berrettini *et al.* [59], as part of a systematic search in 22 multiply affected families found evidence of a susceptibility gene in the pericentromeric region of chromosome 18. Straub *et al.* [70] reported a possible vulnerability locus for bipolar on chromosome 21q22.3. They examined 47 families with bipolar and reported a Lod score of 3.41 in one family at the PFKL locus on chromosome 21q22.3. Five other families also showed small positive Lod scores with PFKL. The authors concluded that the presence of a gene in 21q22.3 predisposes at least one family to BP disorder. A genome search was reported by Coon *et al.* [71]. Eight pedigrees were examined with 328 DNA markers. Of these, four produced Lod scores (assuming homogeneity) of >1, three of these on distal chromosome 5q. Detera-Wadleigh *et al.* [72] reported results of a genome search for a predisposing locus to BP in 21 moderate sized pedigrees. No linkage was found between marker loci on chromosome 2,3,4,7, 9,10p,11p,22 and the pseudoautosomal region at Xpter. More recently, after a genome wide search for loci linked to bipolar affective disorder in the Old Order Amish, Ginns *et al.* [73] reported small positive Lod scores on chromosomes 6, 13 and 15, which require further study (Fig. 1.3).

Trinucleotide repeats in bipolar disorder

In many multiply affected families transmitting bipolar disorder, an earlier age of onset is observed in younger generations. One explanation is ascertainment bias; families with affected members in several generations are more likely to be those with an older age of onset in the upper generations and an early age of onset in lower generations. Early onset in upper generations might reduce fecundity, and a late onset in lower generations might mean the demise of the previous generation prior to possible ascertainment. Apparent anticipation might therefore be due to ascertainment bias and regression to the mean. While acknowledging these difficulties McInnis *et al.* [76] have looked at 34 families and concluded that true anticipation existed.

However, allowing for some uncertainty in bipolar disorder, several other neuropsychiatric diseases with true anticipation are known to exist, and furthermore, a molecular mechanism has been identified. Tandemly expanded trinucleotide repeats have been identified as the cause of some of these diseases including, most famously, Huntington's disease. It is

Fig. 1.3 *Genome searches in affective disorders. + indicates positive findings but not necessarily significant. – indicates negative findings.*

Genome searches in affective disorders		
Marker/region	**Reference**	**Linkage**
Classic markers	Kidd *et al.*, 1984 [74]	–
Genome, Ch11p	Gerhard *et al.*, 1984 [64]	small + Ch11
2,3,4,7,9,10p,11p 22, Xpter	Detera-Wadleigh *et al.*, 1994 [72]	–
Genome, Ch21q22.3	Straub *et al.*, 1994 [70]	+
4q,9q,19	Ewald *et al.*, 1994 [33]	–
Genome	Berrettini *et al.*, 1991 [75]	–
Genome, Ch18	Berrettini *et al.*, 1994 [59]	+
328 markers/genome	Coon *et al.*, 1993 [71]	small + Ch5
551 markers/genome	Ginns *et al.*, 1996 [73]	small + Ch6,13,15
Genome	Freimer *et al.*, 1996 [62]	+ Ch18

now clear that these expansions may disrupt a gene even if they are intronic; an expanded intronic GAA repeat has recently been shown to cause Friedreich's ataxia.

A method of repeat expansion detection (RED) has been developed [77], but it is only capable of detecting their existence, and not their location. Evidence to support the presence of trinucleotide expansions somewhere in the genome of manic depressives has been described by O'Donovan *et al.* [78], but attempts to identify specific loci have so far not been successful.

Summary

Several studies report results suggesting either linkage or association in bipolar affective disorders, but none are conclusive. However, some findings appear to have been independently replicated. The chromosome 18 results are very promising, although the region of interest is extremely large. In addition, the evidence for excess expanded trinucleotide repeats has been found in unrelated patients, although not, paradoxically it would appear, in the pedigrees in which anticipation was found. The linkage studies to date have used large pedigrees and are expected to detect major genes if they exist, and then only if they contribute to the disease in most families. Rare single gene subtypes of the disorder may exist. Large family datasets are now coming on line, some consisting only of affected sibling pairs. Genome scans using these resources should identify the location of susceptibility genes (genes of minor effect). Association studies have examined available candidate genes using the case control design; however, as with most linkage studies, suggestive findings have not been replicated. The psychiatric disorders are a difficult area for the application of molecular genetic techniques because of *inter alia* diagnostic uncertainty, the question of the definition of phenotype, unknown mode of inheritance, and probable incomplete or variable expression of susceptible genotypes. Clearly, if major genes do not play a role in the genetic susceptibility to bipolar disorder then large samples will be needed to detect more minor susceptibility genes. As shown recently by Kruglyak and Lander [79], if a mutation contributes to susceptibility to bipolar disorder such that possession of the mutation increases the relative risk to 2, then more than 700 affected sib-pairs will be required for its detection. Such sample sizes will probably be available in the near future.

References

1. Leonhard K: *The Classification of Endogenous Psychoses.* Edited by Robins E. Translation by Berman R. New York: Irvington; 1979.

2. Perris C: **A study of bipolar (manic-depressive) and unipolar recurrent depressive psychoses.** *Acta Psychiatr Scand Suppl* 1966, **194**:1–189.

3. Angst J: *Zur Aetiologie und Nosologie endogener depressiver Psychosen.* Berlin: Springer; 1966.

4. Wing JK, Babor T, Brugha T *et al.*: **SCAN: Schedules for clinical assessment in neuropsychiatry.** *Arch Gen Psychiatry* 1990; **47**:589–592.

5. Mitchell P, MacKinnon A, Waters B: **The genetics of bipolar disorder.** *Aust N Z J Psychiatry* 1993, **27**:560–580.

6. Weissman M, Gershon E, Kidd K, *et al.*: **Psychiatric disorders in the relatives of probands with affective disorders.** *Arch Gen Psychiatry* 1984, **41**:13–21.

7. Blacker D, Tsuang MT: **Unipolar relatives in bipolar pedigrees: are they bipolar.** *Psychiatr Gen* 1993, **3**:5–16.

8. Bertelsen A, Harvald B, Hauge M: **A Danish twin study**

of **manic-depressive disorders.** *Br J Psychiatry* 1977, **130**:330–351.

9. Bertelsen A, Gottesman II: **Offspring of twin pairs discordant for psychiatric illness.** *Acta Genet Med Gemellol* 1986; **35**:310.

10. Mendlewicz J, Rainer J: **Adoption study supporting genetic transmission in manic depressive illness.** *Nature* 1977, **268**:327–329.

11. Morton NE: *Outline of Genetic Epidemiology.* Basel: Karger; 1982.

12. Goate A, Charter-Harlin M, Mullan M, *et al.*: **Segregation of a missense mutation in the amyloid precursor protein gene with familial Alzheimer's disease.** *Nature* 1991, **349**:704–706.

13. Lyonnet S, Bolino A, Pelet, *et al.*: **A gene for Hirschsprung disease (megacolon) in the pericentromeric region of human chromosome 10.** *Natural Genet* 1993, **4**:346–351.

14. Joutel A, Bousser M-G, Biousse V, *et al.*: **A gene for familial hemiplegic migraine maps to chromosome 19.** *Nature Genet* 1993, **5**:40–45.

15. Poirier J, Davignon J, Bouthilier D, *et al.*: **Apolipoprotein E polymorphism and Alzheimer's disease.** *Lancet* 1993, **342**:697–699.

16. Davies JL, Kawaguchi Y, Bennett S, *et al.*: **A genome-wide search for human type 1 diabetes susceptibility genes.** *Nature* 1994, **371**:130–136.

17. Morton NE: **Sequential tests for the detection of linkage.** *Am J Hum Genet* 1955, **7**:277–318.

18. Penrose L: **The general purpose sib-pair test.** *Ann Eugenics* 1953, **6**:133–138.

19. Thompson G: **Determining the mode of inheritance of RFLP-associated diseases using the affected sib-pair method.** *Am J Hum Genet* 1986, **39**:207–221.

20. Leboyer M, Malafosse A, Boularand S, *et al.*: **Tyrosine hydroxylase polymorphisms associated with manic depressive illness.** *Lancet* 1990, **335**:1219

21. Mitchell P, Selbie L, Waters B, *et al.*: **Exclusion of close linkage of bipolar disorder to dopamine D1 and D2 receptor gene markers.** *J Affective Disord* 1992, **25**: 1–12.

22. Byerley W, Leppert M, O'Connell P, *et al.*: **D2 Dopamine receptor gene not linked to manic-depression in three families.** *Psychiatr Genet* 1990, **1**:55–62.

23. Mitchell P, Waters B, Vivero C, *et al.*: **Exclusion of close linkage of bipolar disorder to the Dopamine D3 receptor gene in nine Australian pedigrees.** *J Affective Disord* 1993, **27**:213–224.

24. Shaikh S, Ball D, Craddock N, *et al.*: **The dopamine D3 receptor gene: no association with bipolar affective disorder.** *J Med Genet* 1993, **30**:308–309.

25. Nanko S, Fukuda R, Hattori M, *et al.*: **Linkage studies between affective disorder and dopamine D2, D3 and D4 receptor gene loci in four Japanese pedigrees.** *Psychiatry Res* 1994, **52**:149–157.

26. Lim LCC, Nothen MM, Korner J, *et al.*: **No evidence of association between dopamine D4 receptor variants and bipolar affective disorder.** *Am J Med Gen* 1994, **54**: 259–263.

27. Sherrington R, Brynjolfsson J, Curtis D, *et al.*: **A linkage study with the D5 dopamine receptor in Icelandic pedigrees with multiple cases of manic depression.** *Psychiatr Genet* 1993, **3**:241–245.

28. Byerley W, Hoff M, Holik J, *et al.*: **Linkage study with D5 Dopamine and alpha(2c)-adrenergic receptor genes in six multiplex bipolar pedigrees.** *Psychiatr Genet* 1994, **4**:121–124.

29. De Bruyn A, Mendelbaum K, Sandkuijl LA, *et al.*: **Non-linkage of bipolar illness to tyrosine hydroxylase, tyrosinase and D2 and D4 dopamine receptor genes on chromosome 11.** *Am J Psychiatry* 1994, **151**:102–106.

30. Lim LCC, Gurling H, Curtis D, *et al.*: **Linkage between tyrosine hydroxylase gene and affective disorders cannot be excluded in two of six pedigrees.** *Am J Med Genet* 1993, **48**:223–228.

31. Sidenberg DG, King N, Kennedy JL: **Analysis of new D4 dopamine receptor (DRD4) coding region variants and TH microsatellite in the Old Order Amish family (00A110).** *Psychiatric Genet* 1994, **4**:95–99.

32. Lim LCC, Powell JF, Murray R, *et al.*: **Monoamine oxidase A gene and bipolar affective disorder.** *Am J Hum Genet* 1994, **54**:1122–1124.

33. Ewald H, Mors O, Flint F, *et al.*: **Linkage analysis between manic depressive illness and the dopamine beta-hydroxylase gene.** *Psychiatr Genet* 1994, **4**: 177–183.

34. Todd R, O'Malley K: **Population frequencies of tyrosine hydroxylase restriction fragment length polymorphisms in bipolar affective disorder.** *Biol Psychiatry* 1989, **25**:626–630.

35. Nothen M, Korner J, Lanczik M, *et al.*: **Tyrosine hydroxylase polymorphism and manic depressive illness.** *Lancet* 1990, **336**:575.

36. Gill M, Castle D, Hunt N: **Tyrosine hydroxylase polymorphism and bipolar affective disorder.** *J Psychiatric Research* 1991, **25**:179–184.

37. Korner J, Rietschel M, Hunt N, *et al.*: **Association and haplotype analysis at the tyrosine hydroxylase locus in a combined German-British sample of manic depressive patients and controls.** *Psychiatric Genet* 1994, **4**: 167–175.

38. Byerley W, Plaetke R, Hoff M, *et al.*: **Tyrosine hydroxylase gene not linked to manic depression in seven of eight pedigrees.** *Hum Hereditary* 1992, **42**:259–263.

39. Dawson E, Parfitt E, Roberts Q, *et al.*: **Linkage studies of bipolar disorder in the region of the Darier's disease gene on chromosome 12q23-24.** *Am J Med Genet (Neuropsychiatr Genet)* 1994, **60**:94–102.

40. Egeland J, Gershad D, Pauls D, *et al.*: **Bipolar affective disorders linked to DNA markers on chromosome 11.** *Nature* 1987, **325**:783–787.

41. Korner J, Fritze J, Propping P: **RFLP alleles at the tyrosine hydroxylase locus: No association found to affective disorders.** *Psychiatry Res* 1990, **33**:275–280.

42. Mendlewicz J, Verbanck P, Linkowski P, *et al.*: **HLA antigens in affective disorders and schizophrenia.** *J Affective Disord* 1981, **3**:17–24.

43. Holmes D, Brynjolfsson J, Butt P, *et al.*: **No evidence for a susceptibility locus predisposing to manic depression in the region of the dopamine (D2) receptor gene.** *Br J Psychiatry* 1992, **125**:35–39.

44. Rietschel M, Nothen MM, Lannfelt L, *et al.*: **A serine to glycine substitution at position 9 in the extracellular N-terminal part of the dopamine D3 receptor protein — No role in the genetic predisposition to bipolar affective disorder.** *Psychiatry Res* 1993, **46**:253–259.

45. Perez De, Casto, I, Torres P, *et al.*: **No association between dopamine D4 receptor polymorphism and**

manic depressive illness. *J Med Genet* 1994, **31**: 897–898.

46. Craddock N, Owen M, Burge S, *et al.*: **Familial cosegregation of major affective disorder and Darier's disease (Keratosis follicularis).** *Br J Psychiatry* 1994, **164**: 355–358.

47. Craddock N, Dawson E, Burge S, *et al.*: **The gene for Darier's disease maps to chromosome 12q23–q24.1.** *Hum Molec Genet* 1993, **2**:1941–1943.

48. Mendlewicz J, Fleiss J, Fieve R: **Evidence for X-linkage in the linkage in the transmission of manic depressive illness.** *JAMA* 1972, **222**:1624–1627.

49. Mendlewicz J, Fleiss J: **Linkage studies with X-chromosome markers in bipolar and unipolar illness.** *Biol Psychiatry* 1974, **9**:261–294.

50. Mendlewicz J, Linkovski P, Wilmotte J: **Linkage between glucose 6 phosphate dehydrogenase deficiency and manic depressive psychosis.** *Br J Psychiatry* 1980, **137**:337–343.

51. Gershon ES, Targum SD, Matthysse S, *et al.*: **Colour blindness not closely linked to bipolar illness.** *Arch Gen Psychiatry* 1979, **36**:1423–1430.

52. Gejman PV, Detera-Wadleigh S, Martinez MM, *et al.*: **Manic depressive illness not linked to factor IX region in an independent series of pedigrees.** *Genomics* 1990, **8**:648–655.

53. Baron M, Risch N, Hamburger R, *et al.*: **Genetic linkage between X-chromosome markers and bipolar affective illness.** *Nature* 1987, **326**:289–292.

54. Mendlewicz J, Simon P, Sevy S, *et al.*: **Polymorphic DNA marker on X chromosome and manic depression.** *Lancet* 1987, **ii**:1230–1231.

55. Gill M, Castle D, Duggar C: **Cosegregation of Christmas disease and major affective disorder in a pedigree.** *Br J Psychiatry* 1992, **160**:112–114.

56. Lucotte G, Landoulsi A, Berriche S, *et al.*: **Manic depressive illness is linked to factor IX in a French pedigree.** *Ann Genet* 1992, **35**:93–95.

57. Baron M, Freimer NF, Risch N, *et al.*: **Diminished support for linkage between manic depressive illness and X-chromosome markers in three Israeli pedigrees.** *Nature Genet* 1993, **3**:49–55.

58. Hebebrand J: **A critical appraisal of X-linked bipolar illness:evidence for the assumed mode of inheritance is lacking.** *Br J Psychiatry* 1992, **160**:7–11.

59. Berrettini WH, Ferraro TH, Goldin LR, *et al.*: **Chromosome 18 DNA markers and manic-depressive illness: Evidence for a susceptibility gene.** *Proc Nat Acad Sci U S A* 1994, **91**:5918–5921.

60. DeBruyn A, Souery D, Mendelbaum K, *et al.*: **Linkage analysis of families with bipolar illness and chromosome 18 markers.** *Biological Psychiatry* 1996, **39**:679–688.

61. Pauls DL, Ott J, Paul SM, *et al.*: **Linkage analyses of chromosome 18 markers do not identify a major susceptibility locus for bipolar affective disorder in the Old Order Amish.** *Am J Hum Genet* 1995, **57**:636–643.

62. Freimer N, Reus V, Escamilla M, *et al.*: **Genetic mapping using haplotype, association and linkage methods suggests a locus for sever bipolar disorder (BP) at 18q22-q23.** *Nature Genet* 1996, **12**:436–441.

63. Blackwood D, He L, Morris S, *et al.*: **A locus for bipolar affective disorder on chromosome 4p.** *Nature Genetics* 1996, **12**:427–430.

64. Gerhard DS, Egeland JA, Pauls DL, *et al.*: **Is a gene for affective disorder located on the short arm of chromosome 11?** *Am J Hum Genet* 1984, **36**:3S.

65. Detera-Wadleigh SD, Berrettini WH, Goldin LR, *et al.*: **Close linkage of c-Harvey-ras-1 and the insulin gene to affective disorder is ruled out in three North American pedigrees.** *Nature* 1987, **325**:806–808.

66. Gill M, McKeon P, Humphries P: **Linkage analysis of manic depression in an Irish family using H-ras 1 and INS DNA markers.** *J Med Genet* 1988, **25**:634–635.

67. Hodgkinson S, Sherrington R, Gurlling H, *et al.*: **Molecular genetic evidence for heterogeneity in manic depression.** *Nature* 1987, **325**:805–806.

68. Watt DC, Edwards J: **Caution in location the gene(s) for affective disorder.** *Psychol Med* 1989, **19**:273–275.

69. Kelsoe J, Ginus E, Egeland J, *et al.*: **Re-evaluation of the linkage relationship between chromosome 11p loci and the gene for bipolar affective disorder in the Old Order Amish.** *Nature* 1989, **342**:238–243.

70. Straub R, Lehner T, Luo Ying, *et al.*: **A possible vulnerability locus for bipolar affective disorder on chromosome 21q22.3.** *Nature Genet* 1994, **8**:291–296.

71. Coon J, Jensen S, Hoff M, *et al.*: **A genome-wide search for genes predisposing to manic depression, assuming autosomal dominant inheritance.** *Am J Hum Genet* 1993, **52**:1234–1249.

72. Detera-Wadleigh SD, Hsieh WT, *et al.*: **Genetic linkage mapping for a susceptibility locus to bipolar illness: Chromosome 2,3,4,7,9,10p,11p,22 and Xpter.** *Am J Med Genet* 1994, **54**:206–218.

73. Ginns E, Ott J, Egeland J, *et al.*: **A genome-wide search for chromosomal loci linked to bipolar affective disorder in the Old Order Amish.** *Nature Genet* 1996, **12**:431–435.

74. Kidd KK, Egeland J, Molthan L, *et al.*: **Amish study IV: Genetic linkage study of pedigrees of bipolar probands.** *Am J Psychiatry* 1984, **141**:1042–1048.

75. Berrettini WH, Detera-Wadleigh SD, Goldin LR, *et al.*: **Genomic screening for genes predisposing to bipolar disease.** *Psychiatr Genet* 1991, **2**:192–208.

76. McInnis M, McMahon J, Chase G, *et al.*: **Anticipation in bipolar affective disorder.** *Am J Hum Genet* 1993, **53**: 385–390.

77. Schalling M, Hudson T, Buetow K, *et al.*: **Direct detection of novel expanded trinucleotide repeats in the human genome.** *Nature Genet* 1993, **4**:135–139.

78. O'Donovan M, Owen M, Craddock N, *et al.*: **Expanded CAG repeats in schizophrenia and bipolar disorder.** *Nature Genetics* 1995, **10**:380–381.

79. Kruglyak L, Lander E: **High-resolution genetic mapping of complex traits.** *Am J Hum Gen* 1995, **56**:1212–1223.

2

Neurochemistry and neuropharmacology

Lucinda Scott and Timothy G. Dinan

Introduction

This chapter will describe the synthesis, anatomy, physiology and receptor systems of acetylcholine and the major biogenic amines, noradrenaline, dopamine and serotonin as well as the involvement of intracellular messenger systems in the modulation of neurotransmitter function. Glutamate and gamma-aminobutyric acid (GABA), excitatory and inhibitory amino acids, respectively, will be covered in a similiar manner; both have been the subject of considerable interest in the psychiatric literature over the past decade. The peptides have also excited much research interest, this focusing largely on thyrotropin-releasing hormone, vasoactive intestinal peptide, somatostatin, cholecystokinin (CCK) and neurotensin, in addition to the endorphins. Rather than discuss psychotropic drugs in detail this chapter provides a framework of basic neurochemistry and pharmacology for information found elsewhere concerning, for example, the mode of effect and side effect profiles of individual psychotropic agents.

Classic neurotransmitters

A neurotransmitter is a substance released at the synapse of a neurone which attaches to a specific receptor on a second neurone and exerts a specific effect. To be classified as one a substance must be present in nerve endings and be secreted in response to a stimulus. Precursors and enzymes for its synthesis should be available, as should mechanisms for its degradation.

Acetylcholine

Acetylcholine was the first neurotransmitter to be discovered. It is used in the motor neurones of the spinal cord, preganglionic neurones of the autonomic nervous system and in the parasympathetic postganglionic neurones. The main cholinergic pathways are cortical projections (mainly frontal and parietal) from the nucleus basalis of Meynert in the ventromedial globus pallidus, which also has connections to the thalamus, amygdala and hippocampus.

The rate of synthesis of acetylcholine depends on the supply of choline from plasma. Choline acetyl transferase is found in cell bodies and moves along to the synapse by slow axonal transport. Cholinergic neurones recycle choline, that is, they do not reuptake acetylcholine following its release. Choline acetyl transferase, the principal synthetic enzyme, is a more specific marker of cholinergic tracts than acetylcholine esterase, the primary degradatory enzyme. Physostigmine and neostigmine are reversible inhibitors of acetylcholinesterase, whereas organophosphorus inhibitors are irreversible.

Acetyl CoA + Choline

↓ Choline acetyl transferase

Acetylcholine + Coenzyme A

Cholinergic receptors are divided into two main groups: nicotinic and muscarinic. Nicotinic receptors are typically quick, are always excitatory, are blocked by curare and stimulated by nicotine and acetylcholine. These receptors form ligand-gated ion channels. Muscarinic receptors are typically slow, are excitatory or inhibitory, are blocked by atropine and stimulated by muscarine, pilocarpine and arecoline. They are coupled to G proteins. At least five different receptor subtypes exist, the two most important are M1 and M2 [1], both of which act via second messenger systems.

Catecholamines

Dopamine and noradrenaline are synthesized by a common pathway (Fig. 2.1).

L-tyrosine is hydroxylated to L-DOPA (by tyrosine hydroxylase), L-DOPA is decarboxylated to dopamine (by aromatic L-amino acid decarboxylase) and dopamine is then hydroxylated to noradrenaline (by dopamine beta-hydroxylase). The rate-limiting step in the synthesis of noradrenaline and dopamine is the conversion of L-tyrosine to L-DOPA by tyrosine hydroxylase [2]. This step is inhibited by alpha-methyl-paratyrosine. The main break down product of noradrenaline is 3-methoxy-4-hydroxyphenylglycol (MHPG).

Fig. 2.1 *Catecholamines: the synthesis and degradation of dopamine and noradrenaline. COMT, catechol-O-methyltransferase; MAO, monoamine oxidase.*

Cathecholamines: the synthesis and degradation of dopamine and noradrenaline

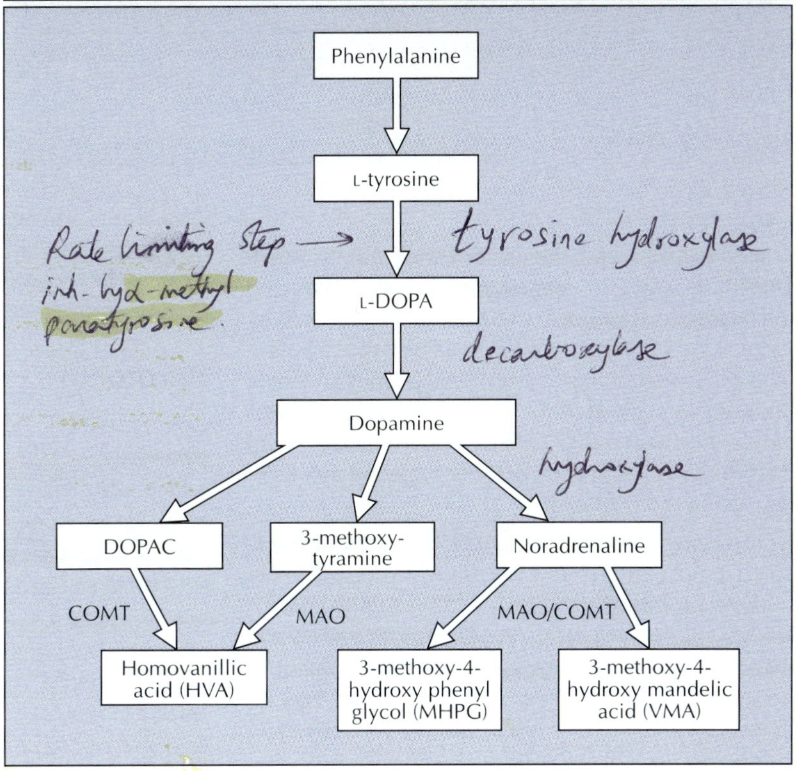

Dopamine is catabolized to homovanillic acid and DOPAC (dihydroxyphenylacetic acid; the deaminated metabolite of dopamine). Two enzymes are concerned in the metabolism of catecholamines, namely monoamine oxidase, which occurs mainly intraneuronally, and catechol-O-methyltransferase which is restricted to the synaptic cleft.

Noradrenaline

The most important noradrenergic projections with regard to psychological function arise from the locus coeruleus, a dense collection of cells found at the floor of the fourth ventricle of the pons. They ascend from the brainstem as the dorsal noradrenergic bundle to innervate the thalamus, hypothalamus, hippocampus and cortex. The ventral noradrenergic bundle arises from medullary collections of neurones and terminates in the hypothalamus and subcortical limbic regions [3].

Early studies of the peripheral sympathetic system established the existence of alpha and beta receptors [4]. Recently, these two major classes of adrenergic receptors have been further subtyped. The alpha-1 receptor, traditionally linked to smooth muscle contraction and glandular secretion, exerts its intracellular effects through a second messenger system, the phosphoinositide system, whereas alpha-2 receptors are coupled to a guanidine triphosphate (GTP)-binding protein, Gi, that inhibits adenylate cyclase.

Beta receptors are also linked to a GTP-binding protein but stimulate adenylate cyclase, Gs, causing an elevation of cyclic adenosine monophosphate (cAMP) and a cascade of intracellular responses. Beta-1 receptors are localized to the heart and in the brain are concentrated in neurones, whereas beta-2 receptors are more localized to glia and blood vessels.

Presynaptic receptors appear to be of both alpha and beta type; stimulation of the alpha-2 receptor inhibits further noradrenaline release, whereas presynaptic beta-receptor stimulation facilitates it. Presynaptic alpha-receptor blockade facilitates, and beta-receptor blockade inhibits, noradrenaline release (Fig. 2.2).

Fig. 2.2 *Adrenergic receptors.*

Adrenergic receptors

	Alpha-1	Alpha-2	Beta-1	Beta-2
Agonist	phenylephrine	clonidine	isoprenaline	salbutamol
Antagonist	prazosin	phentolamine	atenolol	
		yohimbine	← propanolol →	

Dopamine

The three main dopaminergic pathways are the nigrostriatal pathway, the mesolimbic cortical bundle and the tuberoinfundibular system. The former involves projections from the zona compacta of the substantia nigra to the striatum, whereas the latter connects the arcuate nucleus of the hypothalamus to the pituitary. The mesolimbic cortical bundle passes from the ventral tegmental area to innervate the mesolimbic system and cortex [5].

Until the mid-1980s dopamine receptors were classified simply as D_1- and D_2-like receptors. The D_1 receptor is bound by the benzodiazepine antagonist SCH 23390, whereas the D_2 receptor is bound with high affinity by the butyrophenones (haloperidol and spiperone). This classification still stands [6] with other cloned receptors falling into these two categories.

The dopamine D_1-like receptors include D_1 and D_5 and the dopamine D_2-like receptors include D_2, D_3 and D_4. At least 21 different variants of the human D_4 receptor gene exist [7]. D_1 and D_5 are linked to adenylate cyclase by a Gs protein. The D_2, D_3 and D_4 are negatively coupled to adenylate cyclase by Gi.

With regard to distribution, the D_5 receptor appears to be expressed outside the striatum, whereas the D_1 receptor is most abundant in the caudate, nucleus accumbens and the olfactory tubercle with little in the striatum, whereas D_2 receptors are expressed at high levels in the striatum. The D_3 receptor is more narrowly distributed, being found predominantly in limbic areas, such as the hypothalamus, and in the nucleus accumbens. This concentration in the limbic areas suggests that the D_3 receptor may be particularly relevant to the antipsychotic actions brought about by dopamine blockade. The D_3 receptor that is found presynaptically is now believed to function as an autoreceptor [8].

Clozapine is atypically antipsychotic and binds with high affinity to the D_4 receptor which, like D_3, is concentrated in the limbic areas rather than the striatum. This distribution may account for the low incidence of motor side effects experienced with clozapine treatment as extrapyramidal side effects are attributed to D_2-receptor blockade in the striatum.

Serotonin

Serotonin (5HT) is an indoleamine neurotransmitter synthesized from tryptophan (Fig. 2.3), an essential amino acid found in the diet that is preferentially taken up by serotonergic neurones. The rate-limiting step in its formation involves tryptophan hydroxylase. 5HT is catabolized by monoamine oxidase to form 5-hydroxyindolacetic acid. Extracellular 5HT that escapes metabolism is quickly taken up (reuptake) at the presynaptic site into the cytoplasm. Selective serotonin reuptake inhibitors (SSRIs) such as fluoxetine and sertraline, which are used primarily in the treatment of depression, act at this site increasing the availability of 5HT in the synaptic cleft. Reserpine depletes the intracellular stores of 5HT and parachlorophenylalanine (pCPA) inhibits tryptophan hydroxylase resulting in almost complete depletion of 5HT after several days treatment.

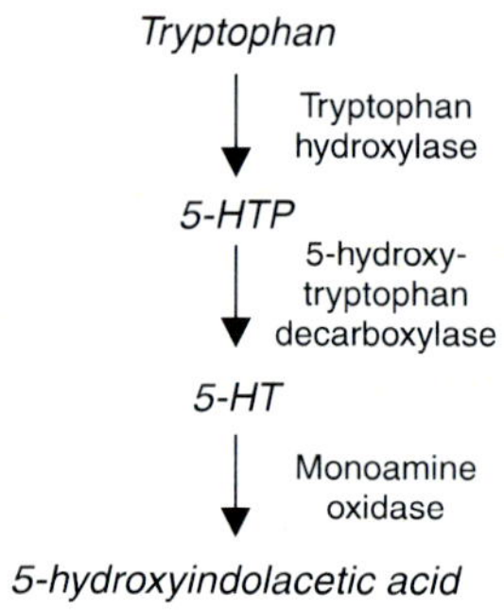

Cell bodies are found in the dorsal and medial raphe nucleus in the pontomedullary region of the brainstem [5]. The major ascending fibres run in the median forebrain bundle and innervate the cerebral cortex, hippocampus, hypothalamus and subcommissural region.

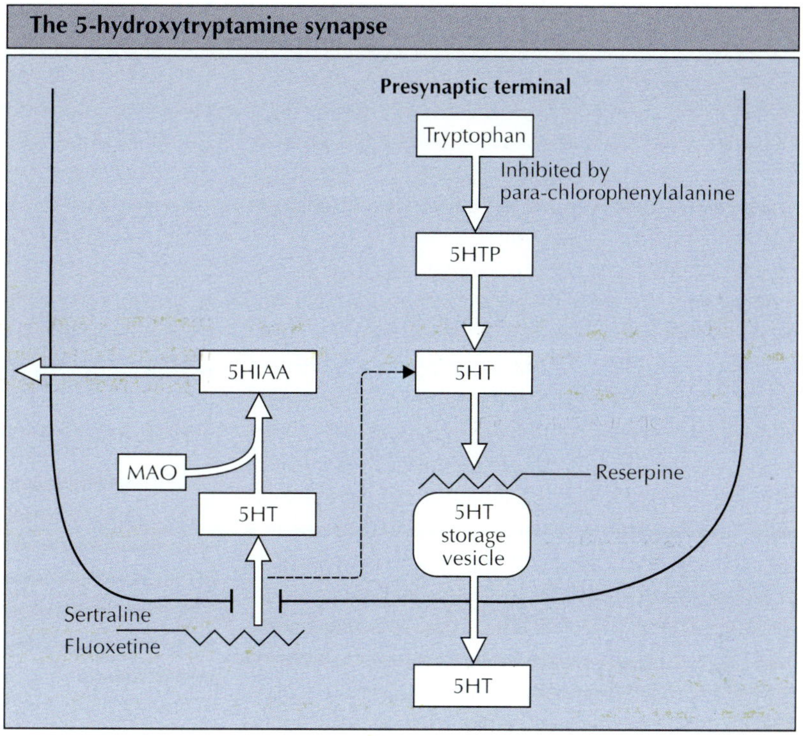

Fig. 2.3 *The 5-hydroxytryptamine pathway. 5HIAA, 5-hydroxyindolacetic acid; 5HT, 5-hydroxytryptamine; 5HTP, 5-hydroxytryptophan; MAO, monoamine oxidase.*

There has been a recent upsurge of interest in 5HT receptor classification to replace that proposed in 1957 by Gaddum and Picarelli [9]. They divided 5HT receptors into D and M types, blocked respectively by dibenzyline and morphine. 5HT receptors are now divided into $5HT_1$, $5HT_2$, $5HT_3$ and $5HT_4$. The $5HT_1$ receptor is further subdivided into 1A, 1B, 1D, 1E and 1F, and the $5HT_2$ receptor into 2A, 2B and 2C [10]. Molecular cloning studies have also revealed the existence of further 5HT receptors for which little pharmacological or physiological data has been found. These include $5HT_{5A}$, $5HT_{5B}$, $5HT_6$ and $5HT_7$. The $5HT_3$ receptor and the nicotinic receptor belong to the family of transmitter-operated ion channels. All other serotonergic receptors act through G proteins.

$5HT_{1A}$ receptor density is highest in the hippocampus and raphe nucleus. Clinically useful drugs that are selective partial agonists at this receptor are buspirone and ipsapirone, both used in the treatment of anxiety. They may owe their activity to an ability to reduce the firing of the raphe nuclei. The $5HT_2$ receptors appear to mediate excitatory effects, most notably in the limbic areas of the brain. $5HT_{2A}$ and $5HT_{2C}$ receptors are concentrated in the medial prefrontal cortex, a region thought to be abnormal in schizophrenia [11]. This and the hallucinogenic properties of LSD and mescaline that are now known to act through the $5HT_2$ receptor provide some of the background for the current interest in the concept of a serotonergic basis for this disorder. The fact that atypical antipsychotic drugs, such as clozapine, bind at the $5HT_2$ receptor has further fuelled this line of investigation.

Excitatory amino acids

Characterization of multiple receptors has led to renewed interest in the role of these agents in the physiological and pathological processes in the central nervous system. L-glutamate is recognized as the major excitatory neurotransmitter in the central nervous system. L-aspartate, cysteic acid and homocysteic acid are also important excitatory amino acids. Glutamate receptors are either ionotropic or metabotropic. The former group is further distinguished by the binding of three agonists: N-methyl-D-aspartate (NMDA), kainate and alpha-amino-3-hydroxy-5-methyl-4-isoxazole propionic acid (AMPA) [12].

NMDA receptor activity is highly regulated by allosteric regulatory binding sites on the receptor–channel complex. These sites are also characterized by voltage-sensitive magnesium blockade. Activation results in long-lasting slow-rising current mediated mainly by influx of calcium. Calcium can mediate longer-lasting cellular responses and forms the basis for long-term potentiation. It does this by triggering a cascade of biochemical events including the production of nitric oxide, which is thought to be the retrograde messenger carrying the long-term potentiation signal. Long-term potentiation is a long-lasting increase in the efficacy of a particular set of synapses brought about by short bursts of high-frequency stimulation which was first described in the hippocampus. It is now thought to be the substrate of associative learning. Blocking of NMDA receptors by a selective antagonist aminophosphonovaleric acid (AP5) not only prevents long-term potentiation but inhibits learning. Overactivation can lead to excessive calcium influx resulting in excitotoxicity and nerve damage. This type of cell death appears to contribute to brain pathology in several conditions including epilepsy and ischaemia [13]. Lamotrigine, the anticonvulsant, works through inhibiting the release of excitatory amino acids, principally glutamate. NMDA receptors usually co-exist with either of the non-NMDA AMPA or kainate receptors. NMDA-receptor subtypes have recently been cloned and include two families of subunits, NMDA1 and NMDA2. They can also be divided on the basis of agonist- or antagonist-preferring properties. Agonist-preferring sites are found for example in the medial striatum whereas antagonist-preferring sites are found in the medial thalamus. Glycine must bind to the receptor–channel complex for the NMDA channel to be activated.

Kainate and AMPA, the non-NMDA receptors, mediate fast excitatory synaptic transmission and are associated mainly with voltage-independent sodium channels. A new class of compounds, 2,3-benzodiazepines, non-competitively block both receptors and have been shown to attenuate ischaemic neuronal injury potently in animals models (Fig. 2.4).

Metabotropic glutamate receptors act via a G protein on second messenger systems. The six metabotropic glutamate receptor subtypes have been classified into three subgroups. Subgroup 1 elicits the release of calcium from intracellular stores acting via a G protein linked to a phosphatidylinositol system. This cascade also involves phospholipase C and protein kinase C. Stimulation of subgroups 2 and 3 causes inhibition of adenylate cyclase with a subsequent reduction in cAMP levels. Induction of long-term potentiation in the hippocampus requires activation of glutamate metabotropic receptors [14].

Inhibitory amino acids

GABA is the main cortical inhibitory neurotransmitter [15]. GABA is found in highest concentrations in the substantia nigra, the globus pallidus and hypothalamus. The Purkinje cells of the cerebellum and some inhibitory interneurones of the spinal cord also use GABA as their transmitter. GABA is synthesized from glutamate via the GABA shunt in a reaction requiring glutamic acid decarboxylase. GABA A receptors are ubiquitous throughout the brain. They form a ligand-gated chloride ion channel complex. GABA B receptors are linked to calcium and potassium channels and are coupled to G proteins. Benzodiazepines bind with high affinity to the GABA A receptor, altering the configuration of the receptor such that the chloride ion channel remains open for longer, thereby potentiating the inhibitory effects of the transmitter. The beta-carbolines, inverse benzodiazepine receptor agonists, are convulsant and decrease rather than increase the effects of GABA. Picrotoxin, which has a binding site on the GABA receptor, is epileptogenic because of its blockade of the chloride channel. Bicuculline is another selective GABA antagonist, whereas baclofen is a selective agonist working through the GABA B receptor system. The GABA B receptor, although less widely distributed than GABA

Glutamate receptors

Type	Bind to	Method of action
Inotropic	NMDA Kainate } non-NMDA receptors AMPA }	Ligand-gated ion channels that regulate ion flux through associated voltage-independent sodium channels
Metabotropic	Subgroup 1,2,3	G protein-coupled receptors which are associated with second messenger systems

Fig. 2.4 *Glutamate receptors. AMPA, alpha-amino-3-hydroxy-5-methyl-4-isoxazole propionic acid; NMDA, N-methyl-D-aspartate.*

A, serves a major role in modulating calcium-dependent neurotransmitter release [16].

Dysfunction of the GABAergic system is thought to contribute to the pathophysiology of convulsive disorders, and many anticonvulsants reinforce GABA-ergic neurotransmission. Gabapentin, the anticonvulsant, was designed to cross the blood–brain barrier as GABA itself does not cross the blood–brain barrier in sufficient amounts. Gabapentin is an effective antiepileptic with low toxicity.

Glycine, the second most important inhibitory neurotransmitter produces its effect by hyperpolarizing the nerve membrane through increased permeability to chloride ions. The receptor which is found post-synaptically is part of the 'ligand-gated superfamily of receptors' [17]. Serine is its major metabolic precursor. Its main action is to mediate inhibition in the spinal cord and brainstem. Strychnine is a potent antagonist. The amino acids taurine and beta-alanine have agonistic properties at the glycine receptor.

Peptides

Peptide transmitters and cotransmitters are different from the classic neurotransmitters in the following ways. Neurotransmitters produce their effect in nanomolar or micromolar concentrations, whereas peptides work in picomolar concentrations. The rate of synthesis of peptides is probably lower. Neurotransmitters bind to their receptors with high affinity but low potency whereas peptides bind with low affinity but high potency. The following are some examples of what is an ever enlarging number of neuropeptides: endorphins, somatostatin, vasoactive intestinal peptide, CCK, neurotensin, thyrotropin-releasing hormone, corticotropin-releasing hormone, substance P, bombesin and angiotensin. The first five will be discussed in more detail below. In mammalian and human brain acetylcholine has been found to colocalize with vasoactive intestinal peptide, dopamine with CCK-8-like peptide and 5HT with substance P. Somatostatin, neurotensin, thyrotropin-releasing hormone and corticotropin-releasing hormone are all peptides found in the hypothalamus. They are implicated as chemical mediators in a variety of pathways subserving thermoregulation, sleep, pain and responses to stress.

Endorphins

Three distinct families of endogenous opiates have been identified: the enkephalins, endorphins and dynorphins. They are derived from distinct precursor polypeptides: proenkephalins, pro-opiomelanocortin and prodynorphin. Of note, pro-opiomelanocortin also contains the amino acid sequence for melanocyte-stimulating hormone, ACTH and beta-lipotropin. Three major classes of opioid receptors are found in the central nervous system, designated mu, kappa and delta. Subtypes of each are also likely to exist [18]. Opioids have been shown to bind to another class of receptor, the sigma receptor. Sigma is now known, however, to represent a site associated with the NMDA type of excitatory amino acid receptor, rather than with the pharmacological activity of opioid analgesics.

The highest concentration of opioid receptors appear in the sensory, limbic and hypothalamic regions of the brain. The periaqueductal grey matter and amygdala are particularly heavily endowed. The receptors all facilitate inhibitory neurotransmission in the brain and the gastrointestinal tract. The release of other neurotransmitters and peptides (such as dopamine, acetylcholine, 5HT and corticotropin-releasing hormone) are inhibited. They all appear to be coupled to G proteins and mu and delta receptors appear to operate potassium channels and adenylate cyclase systems while kappa inhibits voltage-dependent calcium channels. The endogenous opioid peptides have a range of affinities for the different types of opioid receptor.

beta-endorphin	mu > delta > kappa
proenkephalin	delta > mu > kappa
dynorphin	kappa > mu > delta

Naloxone, although antagonistic at each of the receptor types, operates principally through the mu receptor and is involved in the dependence related to most of the opioid substances of abuse.

Somatostatin

Somatostatin is a tetradecapeptide that was first isolated from ovine hypothalamus [19]. It is found in high concentrations in the cerebral cortex, hippocampus, hypothalamus and other areas of the limbic system. Iontophoresis of somatostatin produces an inhibitory effect on most brain areas except the pyramidal cells of the hippocampus where it is excitatory. Decreased levels are found in patients with Alzheimer's disease and Parkinson's disease with dementia. Somatostatin plays a role in antinociception possibly by inhibiting substance P release. At a pituitary level it exerts tonic inhibitory control over growth hormone release.

Vasoactive intestinal peptide

This 28 amino acid peptide was originally isolated from porcine intestine. Vasoactive intestinal peptide is found in the gastrointestinal and respiratory tract and in autonomic ganglia. In the central nervous system it is found in high concentrations in the cerebral cortex, hippocampus, amygdala and hypothalamus. It has a potent excitatory effect on neurones in the above areas. Vasoactive intestinal peptide stimulates prolactin, growth hormone, adrenocorticotropic hormone and luteinizing hormone-releasing hormone but has an inhibitory effect on somatostatin release.

Cholecystokinin

CCK is a member of the gastrin family of peptides. It exists in three forms: CCK-8, CCK-33 and CCK-39, the former being the predominant form [20]. It is present in high concentrations in several areas of the central nervous system notably the cerebral cortex, hippocampus and amygdala [21]. CCK-8 has excitatory effects when applied by iontophoresis to neurones in these areas. When administered with morphine, however, it potentiates the inhibitory effect of the dopamine agonist on neurones in the substantia nigra. It co-exists with substance P in the spinal cord and with vasoactive intestinal peptide in the hypothalamus. The two types of CCK receptor are CCK-A and CCK-B. CCK-A sites in the area postrema and in the nucleus tractus solitarius may be associated with vagal afferent projections involved in the cardiovascular and respiratory control mechanisms. Peripherally, CCK plays a role in normal digestion. In the central nervous system its role is less clear but three possibilities are under consideration: modulation of activity on dopamine pathways, inhibition of feeding (satiety) and a role in analgesia. An abnormality of CCK receptors in panic disorder is suggested by the ability of injected CCK agonists to bring about an attack in healthy individuals [22] and also in patients with a history of panic disorder.

Neurotensin

This 13-residue peptide is concentrated in the central hypothalamus and limbic areas where its release is calcium dependent. Neurotensin is variously reported to produce excitatory, inhibitory or no effects on spontaneously firing or glutamate-driven neurones in the central nervous system. Given parenterally it has hypotensive, hypothermic and hyperglycaemic effects in addition to bringing about ACTH release.

New neurotransmitters

Nitric oxide, a labile free radical gas, is now known to act as a neurotransmitter [23]. Carbon monoxide also has neural messenger activity. Nitric oxide is not stored in synaptic vesicles. Instead it is synthesized as needed by nitric oxide synthase from its precursor L-arginine. Nitric oxide is not released by exocytosis into the synaptic cleft, rather it diffuses into adjacent cells. Immunohistochemical staining reveals nitric oxide synthase to be located in the cerebral cortex, hippocampus, striatum and cerebellum. Excess levels of nitric oxide synthase are neurotoxic. Glutamate, produced in excess in response to ischaemic damage, acts via NMDA receptors to stimulate the nitric oxide synthase neurones to produce nitric oxide which diffuses to adjacent neurones producing a toxic effect. Nitric oxide synthase inhibitors may have therapeutic application in treating thrombosis in a fashion similar to the NMDA antagonists mentioned above.

Second messenger systems

Recent studies in neuroscience have shown synaptic neurotransmission to be far more complex a process than was previously thought with the involvement of intracellular messenger systems [24]. These messengers include coupling factors such as G proteins (G proteins are so-called because of their ability to bind guanine nucleotides), second messengers (calcium, cAMP, cGMP, nitric oxide) and the metabolites of phosphatidyl inositol. Together with the phosphorylation of phosphoproteins and protein kinases and their dephosphorylation by protein phosphatases, these messengers mediate the numerous actions of neurotransmitters on their target neurones. Essentially the second messengers activate the second messenger-dependent protein kinases which impact on the 'third messenger', the phosphoproteins, bringing about a diverse range of biological processes. The intracellular messenger systems for some neurotransmitters bring about the opening and closing of ion channels. They also modulate the general metabolic state of the neurone, its ability to synthesize or release neurotransmitter in addition to more long-lasting effects such as the regulation of gene expression in target neurones.

Since the 1960s when the monoamine theory of depression was first muted research in neuroscience and more specifically in biological psychiatry has focused on the monoamines. The development and widespread application of molecular biology techniques in the past decade has broadened our knowledge of brain structure and function, and notably has paved the way to the discovery of almost 1000 peptides. Disentangling the functions and various interactions of these must logically be the next hurdle in the elucidation of brain biology.

References

1. Bonner TI: **The molecular basis of muscarinic receptor diversity.** *Trends Neurosci* 1989, **12**:148–151.

2. Roth RH, Elsworth JD: **Biochemical pharmacology of midbrain dopamine neurones.** In *Psychopharmacology: The Fourth Generation of Progress.* Edited by Meltzer HY. New York: Raven Press; 1995:227–243.

3. Nieuwenhuys R, Voogd J, van Huijzen C: *The Human Central Nervous System.* Berlin: Springer-Verlag.

4. Ahlquist RP: **A study of the adrenotropic receptors.** *Am J Physiol* 1948, **153**:586–600.

5. Dahlstrom A, Fuxe K: **Evidence for existence of monoamine containing neurones in the central nervous system. 1. Demonstration of monoamines in the cell bodies of brain stem neuron.** *Acta Physiol Scand* 1964; **232(suppl)**:1–55.

6. Spano PF, Govoni S, Trabucchi M: **Studies on the pharmacological properties of dopamine receptors in various areas of the central nervous system.** *Adv Biochem Psychopharmacol* 1978, **19**:155–165.

7. Lichter JB, Barr CL, Kennedy JL, *et al.*: **A hypervariable segment in the human dopamine receptor D4 (DRD4) gene.** *Hum Mol Genet* 1993, **2**:767–773.

8. Carlsson A: **Receptor mediated control of dopamine metabolism.** In *Pre- and Post-Synaptic Receptors.* Edited by Usdin E, Bunney WE. New York: Marcel-Dekker; 1975: 40–65.

9. Gaddum JH, Picarelli ZP: **Two kinds of tryptamine receptors.** *Br J Pharmacol* 1957, **12**:325–334.

10. Humphrey PPH, Hartig P, Hoyer D: **A proposed new nomenclature for 5-HT receptors [Review].** *Trends Pharmacol Sci* 1993, **14**:233–236.

11. Weinberger DR: **Implications of normal brain development for the pathogenesis of schizophrenia.** *Arch Gen Psychiatry* 1987; **44**:660–667.

12. Lodge D, Schoepp D: **Excitatory amino acids.** *Trends Pharmacol Sci* Nomenclature Supplement 1993, 4th edn insert.

13. Olney JW: **Excitatory amino acids and neuropsychiatric disorders.** *Biol Psychiatry* 1989, **26**:505–525.

14. Bashir ZI: **Induction of LTP in the hippocampus needs synaptic activation of metabotropic glutamate receptors.** *Nature* 1993, **363**:347–350.

15. Krnjeric K, Schwartz S: **The action of þ-amino-butyric acid on cortical neurones.** *Exp Brain Res* 1967, **3**: 320–336.

16. Bormann J: **Electrophysiology of GABA A and GABA B receptor subtypes.** *Trends Neurosci* 1988, **11**:112–116.

17. Betz H: **Biology and structure of mammalian glycine receptors.** *Trends Neurosci* 1987, **10**:113–117.

18. Wagner JJ, Chavkin CI: **Neuropharmacology of endogenous opioid peptides.** In *Psychopharmacology: The Fourth Generation of Progress.* Edited by Meltzer HY. New York, Raven Press; 1995:519–531.

19. Brazeau P, Vale WL, Burgus R, *et al.*: **Hypothalamic polypeptide that inhibits the secretion of immunoreactive pituitary growth hormone.** *Science* 1973, **179**: 77–79.

20. Dockray GJ, Gregory RA, Hutchinson JB: **Isolation, structure and biological activity of two CCK octapeptides from sheep brain.** *Nature* 1978; **264**:568–570.

21. Beinfeld MC, Meyer DK, Eskay RL, *et al.*: **The distribution of CCK in the central nervous system.** *Brain Res* 1981, **212**:51–57.

22. de Montigny C: **Cholecystokinin tetrapeptide induces panic attacks in healthy volunteers.** *Arch Gen Psychiatry* 1989, **46**:511–517.

23. Bredt DS, Synder SH: **Nitric oxide: a novel neuronal messenger.** *Neuron* 1992, **8**:3–11.

24. Nestler EJ, Hyman SE: **Intraneuronal signaling pathways.** In: *Comprehensive Textbook of Psychiatry, vol 1.* Edited by Kaplan HI, Sadock B. Baltimore: Williams and Wilkins; 1995:52–64.

Neuroimaging

Michael Travis and Lyn Pilowsky

Neuroimaging involves the collection of data related to the central nervous system (CNS) and the display of this information in a form that has a direct relationship to the structure and function of the CNS. Conventionally neuroimaging is divided into structural and functional imaging, but magnetic resonance imaging can give information both on structure and function, and most torms of functional imaging rely on structural information to derive the location of any changes. The use of neuroimaging in psychiatry research has exploded over the past 20 years and many of the findings have distinct implications for the aetiological basis and treatment of psychiatric illness.

Structural imaging

Magnetic resonance imaging (MRI) and computed tomography (CT) are the most widely available and validated methods of structural neuroimaging. Both methods can generate images in the form of a two dimensional 'slice' through the CNS. MRI data can easily be reconstructed in three dimensions, this allows slices to be displayed in any orientation without reorientation of the patient.

Computed tomography

A CT scan is similar to a skull radiograph in that the images depend on the attenuation of X-ray photons through tissue. Attenuation is the slowing and consequent loss of energy of photons as they pass through material of differing densities. Thus the attenuation of the photons depends on the density of the tissue. Low-density areas (i.e. cerebrospinal fluid) appear black because of low attenuation of X-ray photons, this allows almost all the photons to impinge on the X-ray film developing it as black. High-density areas (i.e. bone) appear white. In order to create the detailed structural images seen in CT scans a parallel X-ray tube and X-ray photon detector are rotated around the patient. This gives a series of mini-X-rays with varying attenuations depending on the density of the tissue between the emitter and detector. Using a computer the 'mini-X-rays' are mathematically reconstructed. The image that has become the familiar CT scan is dependent on the X-ray attenuation in a given area as derived from 'mini-X-rays' from different orientations around a plane of the patient. CT scans can be further enhanced by using various contrast media that increase the attenuation of the X-rays in a targeted tissue.

Magnetic resonance imaging

MRI uses a combination of powerful magnets, radiofrequency pulses and the detection of electromagnetic energy in order to produce an image. The patient is placed in a tube surrounded by a powerful magnet (usually about 1.5 Tesla). The strong magnetic field causes the dipole nuclei of any atoms within the field to line up within parallel or anti-parallel arrays and to produce precession. Precession is a cone-like, symmetrical rotation around an axis rather like a spinning gyroscope (Fig. 3.1). The frequency of this rotation is specific to a given nuclear species. Because of the abundance of hydrogen in organic matter, it is the hydrogen nucleus that has the greatest contribution to the magnetic resonance signal. When a radio-frequency impulse is applied, more nuclei move to the higher energy anti-parallel position, a phenomenon known as resonance. The relaxation of the nuclei back to their original position produces electromagnetic energy that is detected as the magnetic resonance signal.

The net magnetization of an object in an external magnetic field can be said to lie in a longitudinal z direction with no magnetization in the transverse xy plane. The application of the radio-frequency impulse changes the net magnetization from direction z to xy (Fig. 3.2). For a given tissue, relaxation in the longitudinal and transverse planes occurs at different rates described by the time constants T-1 and T-2. T-1 denotes relaxation in the longitudinal direction and loss of nuclear energy into the local environment or lattice. T-2 relaxation occurs as a result of 'dephasing' of nuclear precession causing net cancellation of the transverse magnetic vector (spin–spin effect). Generally speaking the higher the fat content of a tissue the shorter both T-1 and T-2 (i.e. for T-1 and T-2, white matter $<$ grey matter $<$ cerebrospinal fluid).

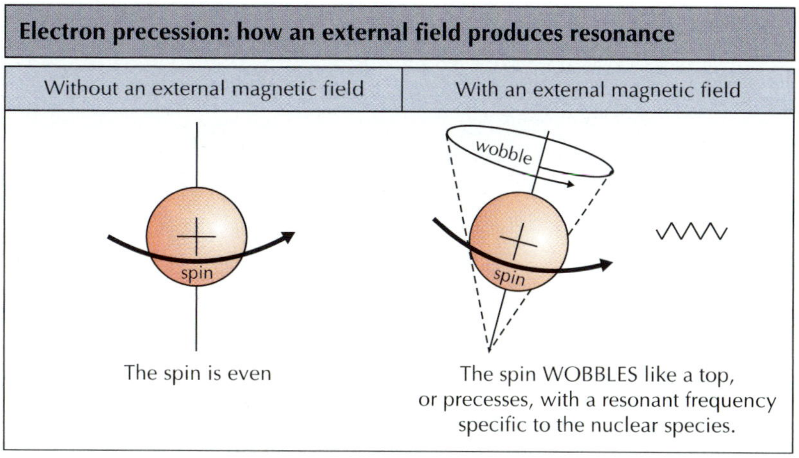

Fig. 3.1 *Electron precession: how an external field produces resonance.*

Manipulation of the radio-frequency impulses allows an image to be T-1 or T-2 weighted. In T-1 weighted images, tissues with short T-1 values give high signal density. In T-2 weighted images tissues with long T-2 values give high signal density. Further manipulation of the radio-frequency impulses allows areas of high proton density (i.e. areas with a high water content) a greater signal. The dynamic nature of an MRI scan implies that any use of magnetic resonance acquires data on the function as well as the structure of the brain.

Clinical uses of CT and MRI structural imaging

CT and MRI structural imaging are primarily used to diagnose organic brain disease by monitoring the progress of chronic disorders and to assess prognosis. A structural scan might be used for patients with focal neurological or cognitive deficit, catatonia or uncharacteristic clinical symptoms (i.e. abrupt personality change or uncommon age of onset). Some centres perform a CT or MRI on all patients with the first onset of psychosis.

MRI has the advantages, over CT, of enhanced resolution and no exposure to ionizing radiation. MRI is also the investigation of choice for white matter lesions (i.e. demyelinating disorder), and when pathology in a specific brain region is suspected and the lesion may be small (i.e. dementia, seizure focus, stroke, vascular malformation, subcortical disorders) (Fig. 3.3).

Although in many ways MRI may seem to be superior to CT, CT scans are more readily available and cheaper. CT should be chosen over MRI when men-

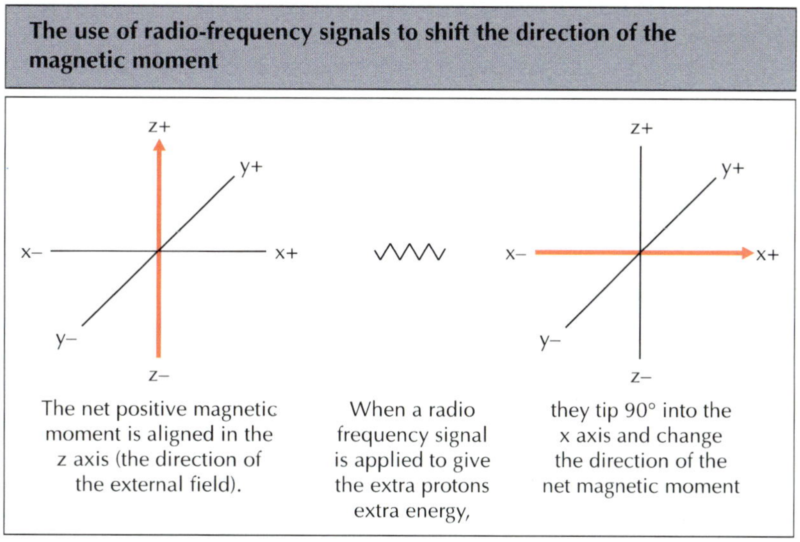

Fig. 3.2 *The use of radio-frequency signals to shift the direction of the magnetic moment. Changes in net magnetization of an object in an external magnetic field after a radio frequency pulse.*

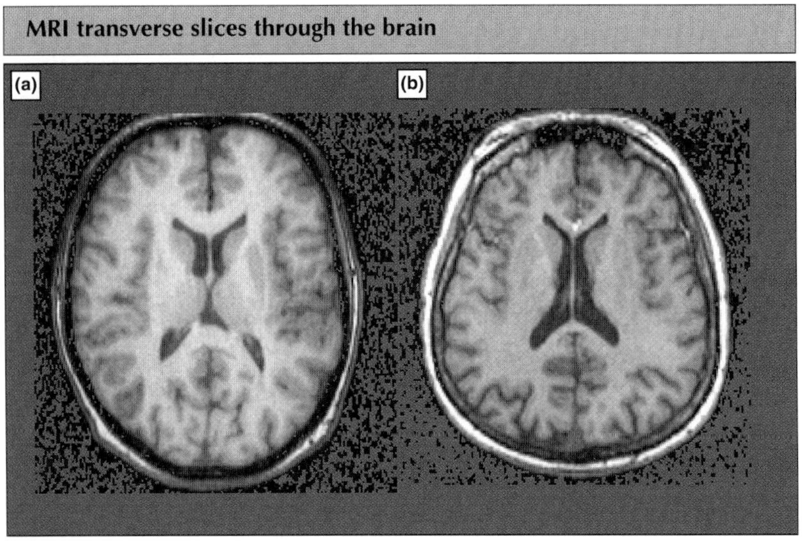

Fig. 3.3 *MRI transverse slices through the brain. (b) Shows a moderate degree of cerebral atrophy. Courtesy of the MRI unit, Maudsley Hospital, London, UK.*

ingeal and pituitary tumours are found or no localizing abnormalities are present. Calcified lesions will also show more clearly on a CT scan. CT may also be used in patients who are unable to have an MRI by virtue of a metallic implant.

Functional imaging

Magnetic resonance imaging

Functional magnetic resonance imaging (fMRI) and magnetic resonance spectroscopy (MRS) are the two techniques whereby the hardware described above is used to generate information about the function and the structure of the brain.

Functional magnetic resonance imaging

fMRI is used for cortical activation mapping. The initial studies in the early 1990s involved tracking repeated bolus doses of an intravenously administered MRI contrast medium, gadolinium [1]. The contrast medium alters the MR signal of water molecules in a complex way. Tracking of the bolus over time allows contrast-enhanced distortions in the magnetic field in each volume segment to be detected. Areas of high blood flow, and therefore activation, lead to a decrease in MR signal density. This method was superseded by the non-invasive blood oxygenation level dependent contrast (BOLD) technique.

Neuronal activity in the brain results in local two- to fourfold changes in cerebral blood flow and volume; however, the use of tissue oxygen only increases slightly. This leads to a relative decrease in deoxyhaemoglobin (containing para-magnetic iron) when compared with oxygenated haemoglobin (containing di-magnetic iron). As this disparity alters the local magnetic field, increased neuronal activity will be reflected by a local enhancement in signal on a T-2 weighted image. This method has the potential pitfall of being unable to account for the volume effect of blood in vessels larger than the capillaries serving the distinct area of the brain activated. This would lead to artifactual areas of activation on the generated image [2].

Application of the recently devised methods of fast MRI acquisition to fMRI has begun to address some of the inadequacies of the previous two methods. Fast low angle shot (FLASH) acquisitions makes use of between 64 and 256 small radio-frequency pulses to excite a small fraction of the equilibrium magnetization, the repetition times of the pulses are far less than the normal relaxation time, T-1. This is combined with a reversal of the external magnetic field gradient between each pulse and allows a very short measuring time. Shorter data acquisition periods can be achieved using rapid reversals of the magnetic field gradient after a single radio-frequency pulse (echoplanar imaging). Echoplanar imaging is up to 20 times faster than FLASH but is more easily affected by magnetic field inhomogeneities.

In relation to the CNS the emphasis is on areas of cortical activation derived from changes in regional cerebral blood flow (rCBF). Activation is seen in the images as changes in signal intensity (Fig. 3.4). The fast acquisition techniques allow discrimination between blood flow effects and regional changes in

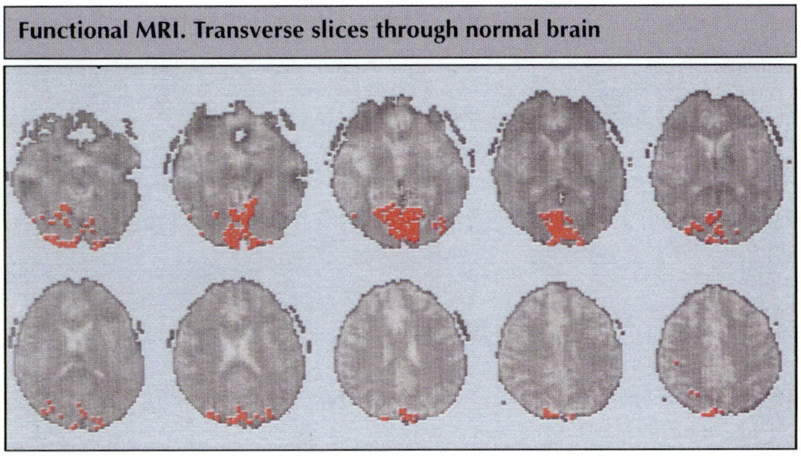

Fig. 3.4 *Functional MRI. Transverse slices through normal brain. The red pixels indicate areas of activation during a visuospatial task. Courtesy of the MRI unit, Maudsley Hospital, London, UK.*

deoxyhaemoglobin concentrations and thus a clearer indication of regional cerebral activation.

Magnetic resonance spectroscopy

MRS differs from MRI and fMRI in that the combination of magnetic field and a series of radiofrequency pulses is used to 'image' nuclei with an odd number of protons and neutrons. After the nuclei line up in the magnetic field, a radiofrequency pulse at the Lamour frequency, which is specific to the nucleus, can cause a given nucleus to absorb and emit energy. The results are usually generated graphically as a series of peaks or as a spectrum where the x-axis is the 'chemical shift' and allows the identification of the nucleus. The height of the peak on the y-axis gives quantitative information about the nucleus of interest. Each individual nucleus behaves differently in different molecules (i.e. the H-1 nucleus in creatinine has a different peak from the H-1 nuclei in choline) because of differences in the electron environment. Therefore a series of peaks for a given nucleus are generated. This gives information about the exact quantity of particular molecules in a given volume of tissue (Fig. 3.5).

Although few applications for MRS (apart from research) are currently available, many different nuclei can be evaluated using this technique. Analysis of fluorine gives information about glucose metabolism and analysis of phosphorous nuclei, i.e. in ATP will give an analysis of bioenergetics. MRS can also be

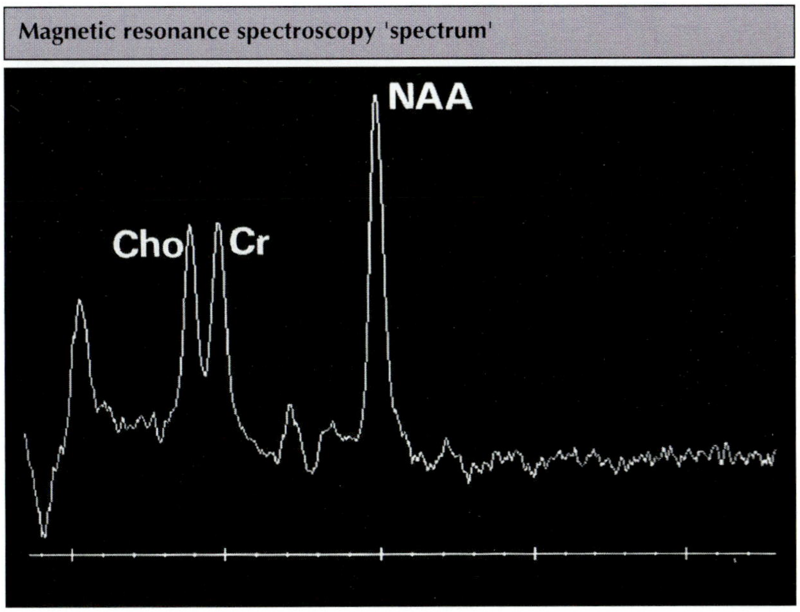

Fig. 3.5 *Magnetic resonance spectoscopy 'spectum'. Cho, peak of choline; Cr, peak of creatinine; NAA, peak of N-acetyl aspartate. Courtesy of the MRI unit, Maudsley Hospital, London, UK.*

used to discover the regional concentration of medications [3].

MRS is a rapidly expanding field and with stronger magnetic fields and more sophisticated computing algorithms it may soon be possible to provide information on individual neurotransmitters *in vivo* without the radioactive isotopes used in positron emission tomography and single photon emission tomography.

Single photon emission (computed) tomography

In single photon emission (computed) tomography [SPE(C)T] a compound labelled with a radioactive isotope emitting gamma photons is given to the patient intravenously, orally or by inhalation. The radiolabelled compound is targeted at a biochemical process or site (e.g. binding to brain receptors, taken up by kidneys or bone). The behaviour of this compound within the patient's organs is then monitored using detectors that allow the emitted gamma photons to be recorded (Fig. 3.6). The compounds used fall into two broad categories. Substances such as HMPAO labelled with technetium-99m are used to measure blood flow in the brain, whereas various receptor ligands, usually labelled with iodine-123, can be used to estimate neuroreceptor number and affinity. Several I^{123}-labelled receptor ligands are readily available for in-vivo imaging in humans. These include iomazenil for the GABA–BDZ (gamma-aminobutyric acid-benzodiazepine), receptor complex (Fig. 3.7), epidipride and IBZM for the dopamine D-2 receptor, and ketanserin for the serotonin receptor [5].

In most brain-dedicated systems two to 12 detectors are arranged around the patient's head. The emitted

The principles of SPET data acquisition

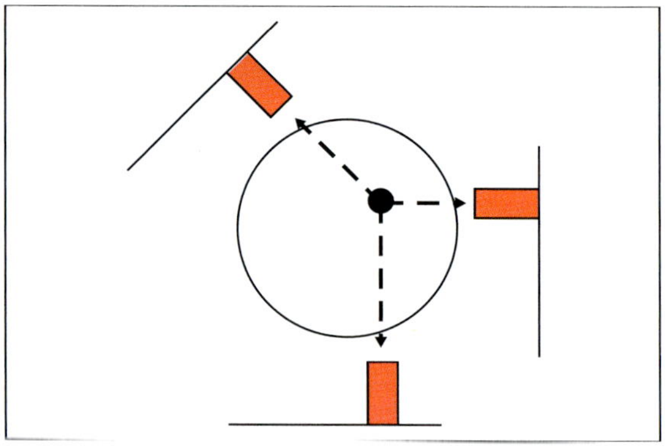

Fig. 3.6 *The principles of SPET data acquisition. The detectors rotate around the object that is emitting gamma photons. Triangulation of the direction of emission allows the placement of the object to be derived. Adapted with permission from [4].*

gamma photons can thus be detected and with the aid of a computer the information can be rendered into a two-dimensional slice or three-dimensional whole brain image that allows regional activities to be calculated [6].

Clinically SPET is relatively cheap and acceptable to patients. SPET has been used to provide a sensitive early measure of cerebral ischaemia before profound structural damage has occurred, i.e. after a transient ischaemic attack. SPET is useful in providing prognostic information after cerebral infarction. As treatments for acute cerebrovascular infarctions are developed, SPET will have a role in determining the site and extent of perfusion deficit. Blood flow and receptor SPET may also have uses in diagnosing Alzheimer's disease [7], and predicting recovery

Typical SPET images

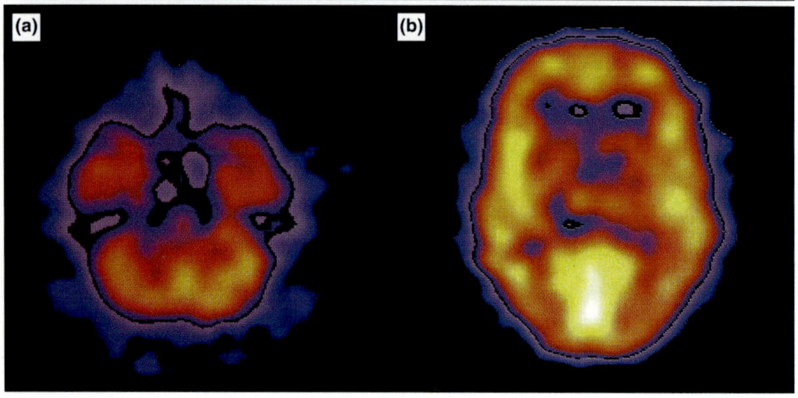

Fig. 3.7 *The images show the distribution of GABA–BDZ receptors in the brain. The brighter the area the greater the number of receptors. The tracer used is I^{123} iomazenil. (a) The cerebellum and inferior temporal lobes. (b) The basal ganglia and occipital cortex. Images courtesy of the Institute of Nuclear Medicine, Middlesex Hospital, London, UK.*

from head injury [8]. Recent SPET receptor studies, using I^{123}-iomazenil, have shown focal lesions in epilepsy patients before surgery [9].

Positron emission tomography

Although the images and functions are similar, positron emission tomography (PET) differs from SPET in several important ways. More labelled tracers are used in PET but the isotopes (most commonly fluorine-18, carbon-11, nitrogen-13 and oxygen-15) have such short half-lives that they must be synthesized in an on-site cyclotron, which makes the individual scans more expensive. The isotopes emit positrons that collide with electrons and thereby produce a pair of gamma photons travelling at 180 degrees to one another (Fig. 3.8). The photons are detected by a ring of detection crystals around the patient's head that are designed to detect the simultaneous arrival of the two particles. Two particles are emitted at a precise angle to one another to allow the computer to provide images with almost twice the resolution of SPET.

The most common tracers used to date include those that measure blood flow ($H_{20}{}^{15}$ and nitrogen^{15}), those that measure metabolic rate (02) and fluorine-18-deoxyglucose, which gives an estimate of the cerebral glucose used. Fluorine^{18} and carbon^{11} have also been used extensively to label receptor ligands with a similar aim to that described for SPET.

PET has few clinical applications. Because using an on-site cyclotron is inconvenient, the technique is available in few centres and is mostly reserved for research studies. There may be future clinical uses for PET similar to those for SPET. The enhanced spatial resolution means that PET can be more easily applied to investigate a suspected functional deficit in a specific area. Several PET and SPET studies have already been conducted using labelled GABA-receptor agonists to seek epileptic foci and dopamine receptor ligands have been used to differentiate and quantify the striatal loss of dopamine receptors in Parkinson's disease [10].

The principles of PET acquisition

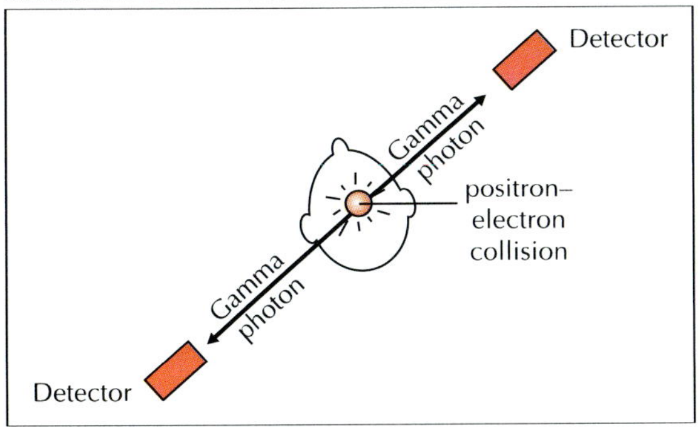

Fig. 3.8 *The principles of PET acquisition. The positron electron collision leads to the coincident emission of two gamma photons at 180 degrees to each other. Only coincident emissions are picked up by the detectors.*

PET and SPET both have lower spatial resolution than magnetic resonance images mainly because of signal attenuation, scatter and partial volume effects; however, both methods are improving rapidly both in the resolution and analysis of images. PET has better spatial resolution than SPET and is the research technique of choice for blood flow activation and localization studies (Fig. 3.9). Recent comparative work [11], however, has indicated that SPET is comparable to PET for receptor imaging. The longer half-life of the [123I] isotope used in SPET over the [11C] isotope used in PET allows the study of ligands with higher receptor affinity and hence a better signal: noise ratio. The shorter half-life of [11C] (20 min versus 13 h for [123I]) means that for highly bound ligands equilibrium between the bound and free fraction of the ligand cannot be reached during the length of a PET study. This prevents the recording of an adequate 'wash-out' phase for these ligands and therefore quantitative analysis of receptors is impossible. This makes SPET the investigation of choice for receptor systems with a low concentration of receptors. These must be studied with high affinity ligands or non-specific, rather than receptor, uptake dominates. New models for the analysis of images are emerging, including the mathematical co-registration of SPET and MRI images. This will allow both SPET and MRI greater anatomical accuracy in regard to regions. Use of mathematical modelling of ligand behaviour will allow more quantitative analysis of receptor parameters.

Neuroimaging and psychiatric disorders

Schizophrenia

When Kraepelin first described 'dementia praecox', he believed it had an organic basis. Unfortunately at the beginning of the century the measuring tools were too crude to point out any distinct brain pathology associated with schizophrenia. By the 1970s

Typical PET scan mapped onto an MRI scan

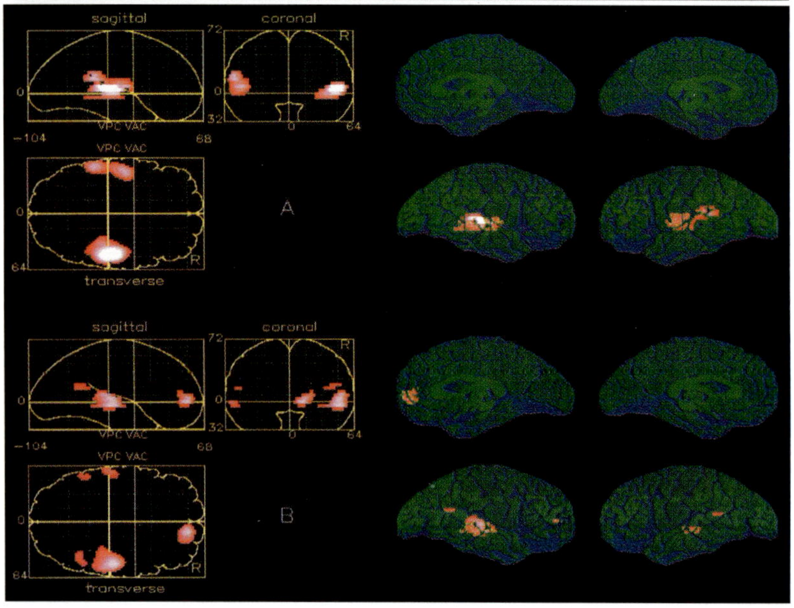

Fig. 3.9 *Typical PET scan mapped onto an MRI scan. The bright areas indicate activation during a speech monitoring task. Courtesy of P. MacGuire, Institute of Psychiatry, London, UK.*

schizophrenia was regarded as the 'graveyard' of neuropathology research. The field of neuroimaging has since contributed hugely to the understanding of schizophrenia and has revitalized the field leading to a number of neuropathological hypotheses.

The most consistent finding in structural imaging studies in schizophrenia is that of lateral ventricular enlargement (up to 62% larger) (Fig. 3.10). This was first noted in pneumoencephalographic investigations in the 1930s and 1950s. This finding was substantiated in the 1970s with CT studies [12], and later replicated using MRI. Increased third and fourth ventricle size has also been demonstrated in schizophrenia. Initial studies used a ventricular brain ratio for a single slice, comparing the size of the ventricles with the rest of the brain tissue in that slice. Later studies measured the volume of the whole ventricle and statistically co-varied for the effects of the whole brain volume. Generally, ventricular enlargement is more pronounced in schizophrenic men than schizophrenic women. The range of ventricular size is usually greater in schizophrenic than control groups. Men tend to have larger lateral ventricles than women in patient and control groups, thus confirming the sexual dimorphic characteristics of this area in common with other brain regions.

Intriguingly, reduced volumes and loss of asymmetry of the structures surrounding the ventricles have also been demonstrated, albeit inconsistently and with little correlation with symptoms. These structures include the amygdala, hippocampus and parahippocampal gyrus. The loss of asymmetry is most marked in the planum temporale, an area which includes the auditory association cortex (Wernicke's area). These areas combined are concerned with selection, association and integration of sensory information, memory and the control of basic drives and emotions, all of which may be disrupted in schizophrenia.

MRI scans taken in coronal section at the level of the posterior bodies of the lateral ventricles

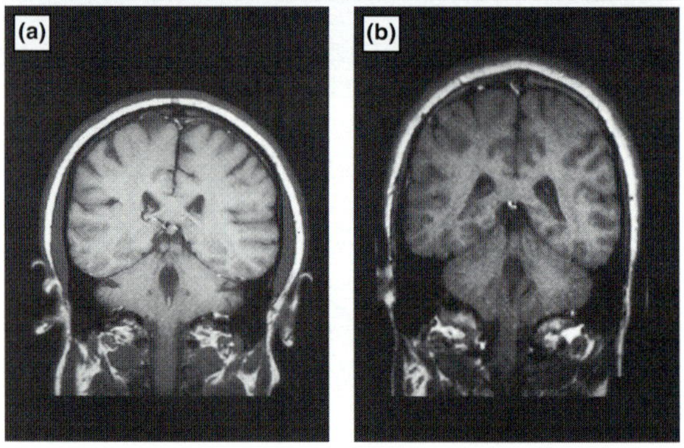

Fig. 3.10 *MRI scans taken in coronal section at the level of the posterior bodies on the lateral ventricles. (a) Healthy volunteer. (b) Age-matched patient with schizophrenia. A typical moderate difference in ventricular size can be seen. Courtesy of P. Woodruff, Institute of Psychiatry, London, UK.*

No relationship exists, however, between duration of illness and structural brain abnormalities; neither do abnormalities progress after symptoms have developed. This has led to the hypothesis that brain abnormalities are not degenerative but long-standing and may represent an incomplete brain maturation or dystrophy of surrounding regions. In studies of discordant monozygotic twins the co-twin unaffected by schizophrenia had smaller ventricles than the affected twin but larger ventricles than twins from unaffected pairs. This would tend to suggest that the increase in ventricular size may be secondary to an acquired environmental factor [13,14].

Functional MRI and MR spectroscopy

Functional magnetic resonance imaging (fMRI) is still in its infancy as a tool in psychiatric research. It has been used extensively for cortical activation mapping, investigating the visual, auditory and motor cortices. Specific functions have also been tested including language function and memory processing. The results of these investigations have confirmed some, but not all, earlier findings from lesion studies and PET and SPET blood flow studies. The increased spatial and temporal resolution of fMRI means that brain blood flow can be viewed with far greater regional accuracy and in real time. Early applications of this technique to schizophrenic patients has indicated that they have an increased response to sensory stimulation and decreased response of the frontal cortex during the performance of cognitive tasks [2].

Magnetic resonance spectroscopy (MRS) has already provided some important insights into brain functioning in schizophrenia. The use of proton MRS has allowed investigation of regional neuronal density. Early studies did not differentiate between patients and healthy individuals. The technique has become more sophisticated and it has become apparent that the reduced mesial temporal volumes seen particularly in schizophrenic men are most likely due to decreased neuronal number. Phosphorus MRS, which gives an estimate of membrane and cell metabolism, has been used more extensively. The first paper in 1991 [15] indicated decreased synthesis and increased breakdown of membrane phospholipids in the dorsolateral prefrontal cortex of schizophrenic patients. This finding has been replicated [16] and may represent a trait marker for schizophrenia that may be more prevalent in negative symptom state [17]. Using MRS, exogenous compounds such as medications can also be studied; however, only early pilot studies have been performed [3].

Positron emission tomography and single photon emission tomography

These studies divide into those examining regional cerebral blood flow and metabolism and those estimating receptor density and function.

Many studies have investigated regional cerebral blood flow (rCBF) and metabolism in schizophrenic patients. Previously, a decrease in frontal blood flow and metabolism (hypofrontality) was believed to indicate schizophrenia; however, some doubt has been cast on these findings [18]. In fact only a minority of studies have found hypofrontality in all schizophrenic patients and a variety of other regional abnormalities have been noted. These include increased rCBF in the left hemisphere and a similar finding in the left globus pallidus. Some studies indicate that the differences in frontal blood flow between patients and control individuals occurred after treatment and others that the changes were persistent. Nevertheless, hypofrontality of blood flow and metabolism is still strongly suggested as a function of deficit schizophrenia. Some activation studies using, for example, the Wisconsin card sorting-test indicated that healthy volunteers have increased blood flow to the dorsolateral prefrontal cortex during the task. This is not apparent when schizophrenic patients perform the task [19]. Again this has proved difficult to replicate and further studies using verbal fluency as an activation found very similar activation patterns in healthy individuals and schizophrenic patients with and without task impairment [20].

Studies of patients attempting to correlate specific symptoms with functional imaging findings have had more success with relatively consistent findings using PET and SPET techniques. Liddle *et al.* [21] defined three symptom clusters: psychomotor poverty, disorganization (i.e. inappropriate affect, speech content abnormalities) and reality distortion (i.e. delusions and hallucinations). They found that reduced rCBF in the left and medial prefrontal cortex correlated with psychomotor poverty, that the severity of disorganization correlated with increased rCBF in the right medial prefrontal cortex and decreased perfusion in Broca's area, and that reality disorientation correlated with increased rCBF in the left hippocampal formation. These findings have subsequently been partially replicated [22]. One SPET study of schizophrenia with and without auditory hallucinations has shown increased blood flow to the Broca's area when patients are hearing voices [23]. More recent studies have implicated the subcortical nuclei in the generation of auditory hallucinations [24,25].

Estimations of receptor density and activity using PET and SPET techniques have to date focused mainly on the dopaminergic system. Virtually all emission tomography studies have found no clear striatal dopamine receptor differences between drug naïve patients and healthy individuals. Subtle alterations including asymmetry of binding have been noted but have not been fully confirmed. In studies of patients on medication, radioactive-labelled ligands have been used to determine the in-vivo receptor occupancy of both typical and atypical antipsychotic drugs, relating these to clinical state. In contrast to the findings in drug-naïve patients emission tomography has partially reinforced the accepted theory that antipsychotic efficacy is related to D2 blockade. Nonetheless the situation appears very complex in that non-responders to antipsychotic drugs may show high levels of striatal D2 blockade. Furthermore the highly effective atypical antipsychotic clozapine produces far less striatal D2 blockade than typical antipsychotics [26,27] (Fig. 3.11). Olanzepine, a recently introduced, clinically effective atypical antipsychotic, has been studied using SPET techniques and has a similarly low striatal D2 receptor occupancy to clozapine [28]. Both clozapine and olanzepine have a low incidence of extra-pyramidal side effects (EPS), and this is no doubt due to the low striatal D2 blockade demonstrated in the functional images. EPS have been the focus of several studies and a putative threshold of 80% D2 occupancy has been suggested to be necessary to produce EPS [29]. An intriguing finding is that risperidone, with similar D2 occupancy, produces far fewer EPS [30]. It has therefore been suggested that the potent $5HT_{2A}$ antagonism of risperidone, also demonstrated by PET, may be protective against EPS.

Affective disorders

Bipolar affective disorder and major depression patients have been studied with a variety of imaging systems. Structural imaging reports of lateral and third ventricular enlargement in affective disorders have been inconsistent and may be related to cognitive changes and cerebral atrophy. Nevertheless, various regions including the caudate, brainstem, vermis and frontal lobe have a reduced volume in depressed patients and this is thought to be due to the high levels of hypercortisolaemia often seen in these patients. Using MRI, deep white matter hyperintensities (DWMH) have been noted to be more frequent in elderly depressed patients compared with age-matched controls. These have also been described as seven times more frequent in young patients with bipolar disorder than healthy controls. The significance of these findings is unclear, but presence of DWMH may be related to cognitive impairment, poorer response to treatment and increased sensitivity to medication and ECT [31].

fMRI has not yet been applied to affective disorders, but MRS has been used, although mainly in bipolar affective disorder patients. These studies have con-

SPET scans acquired using the D_2 ligand I^{123} IBZM

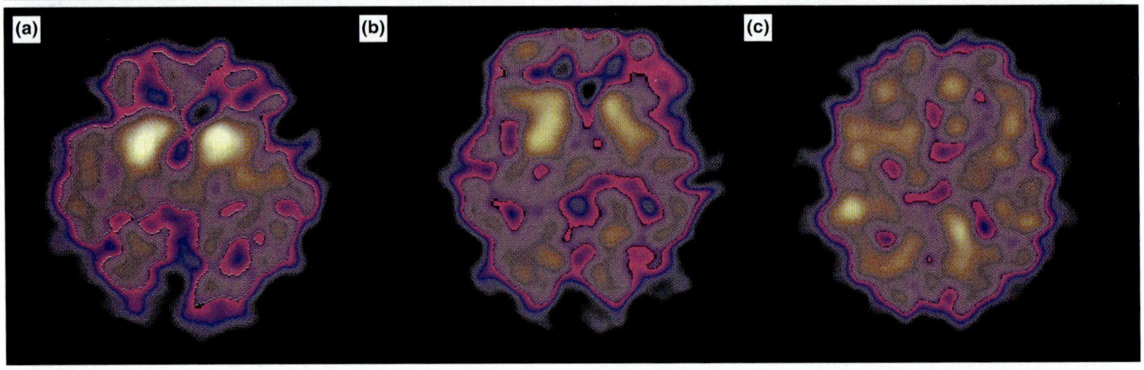

Fig. 3.11 *(a) Striatal dopamine receptors in an untreated schizophrenic patient. (b) The complete blockade of these receptors with a typical antipsychotic drug. (c) The partial blockade of these receptors with an equally efficacious dose of clozapine (an atypical antipsychotic). Images courtesy of Nuclear Medicine, Middlesex Hospital, London, UK.*

sistently shown lower than normal frontal lobe phosphomonoester values in the euthymic state and higher values in both the depressed and manic states. The precise meaning of these abnormalities is unclear but the finding is consistent with the suggestion that lithium acts on phosphorous-containing molecules in cell membranes. MRS has also been used in bipolar patients to investigate the relationship of lithium to treatment response. It was found that improvement in symptoms correlated with lithium concentrations in the brain but not in the plasma [3].

The use of PET and SPET in affective disorders has been limited compared with schizophrenia and the results have been more equivocal. In unipolar depression, some authors [32,33] report a decreased frontal blood flow or metabolism but other results have contradicted these findings. Changes in blood flow and metabolism in the parietal, temporal and anterior cingulate cortices have been reported but these findings tend to vary with the type of depression rather than the severity. Before and after treatment studies have tended to indicate a lower regional blood flow when the patient is depressed compared with the euthymic state [32]. Interestingly, psychomotor retardation is associated with low flow to the dorsolateral prefrontal cortex (DLPFC) in both depression and schizophrenia suggesting that these symptoms may have a common cause. Some authors correlating symptoms with changes in rCBF have suggested that the cognitive errors, such as depressive ruminations and automatic emotional associations, noted in depression are associated with perturbed function in the left ventrolateral prefrontal cortex and that deficits in attention and memory may be linked to decreased rCBF in the bilateral prefrontal cortex and posterior parietal cortex. In addition to this it would appear that the cingulate cortex, an area associated with the mediation and expression of emotion, has reduced blood flow in the depressed state that returns towards normal with clinical recovery, along with the reduced rCBF in the DLPFC [33]. Radiolabelled receptor ligand studies in depressed patients to date have been limited because of a lack of suitable ligands. One SPET study using a 5HT ligand revealed a higher uptake in the parietal cortex of depressed patients compared with healthy individuals and a greater right than left asymmetry in the inferofrontal region [34].

In bipolar patients a decrease in total CBF during the depressed phase has been observed [35]. Other work [36] has described a selective decrease in regional glucose metabolism in the basal ganglia and frontal cortex in bipolar depressives. This work awaits replication.

Anxiety disorders

Structural imaging has added only little to our understanding of most of the anxiety disorders. Findings are often conflicting and few have been replicated. This is with the notable exception of post traumatic stress disorder (PTSD) in which a noted decrease in the size of the right hippocampus correlates with the scores on the Wechsler Memory Scale. This is thought to be due to a relative hypersecretion of cortisol in the early stages of PTSD [37]. Functional imaging has been used extensively to investigate anxiety disorders.

Phobias and panic

MRS has been applied to both panic and social phobic patients. In the phobic group changes were noted in subcortical, thalamic and caudate areas, which ties in with some of the emission tomography work. In panic patients it has been reported that hyperventilation increases brain lactate (also used as an exogenous panic inducer) levels above those seen in healthy individuals with a similar CO_2 washout, this may be due to altered metabolism or a variation in the response of the cerebral circulation to hypocapnia [38].

Emission tomography imaging has revealed differences in regional cerebral blood flow (rCBF) between phobia/panic patients and healthy individuals [39,40]. Areas implicated have included the hippocampi, the occipital, temporal, orbitofrontal and cingulate cortices. The relationship between anxiety and rCBF is complex, however. In healthy individuals Gur *et al.* [41] found that for lower anxiety states an increase in both rCBF and metabolism is found but that as anxiety increased to higher levels these parameters decreased. Receptor ligand studies have so far focused on GABA–BDZ function. Feistel *et al.* [42] found decreased receptor density in the right hippocampus and left temporal region of four patients with panic disorder compared with 10 patients with other disorders, who had a lower score on the Hamilton anxiety scale. In a study of 10 patients with panic disorder. Schlegel *et al.* [43] found lower numbers of BZ receptors in the frontal, occipital and temporal cortices when compared with a matched group of epileptic patients. In contrast to these findings, a more recent study using I^{123} iomazenil SPET demonstrated that, in comparison with healthy individuals, panic patients had an increased right:left ratio of prefrontal cortex tracer uptake and that a trend to increased tracer uptake was found in the temporal regions of panic patients [44]. These disparate findings support the evidence that there are functional cerebral changes in anxiety states that are related to the GABA–BDZ receptor complex. Without a comparison between anxiety disorder groups, however, whether these changes are specific to panic disorder or merely an effect of chronic anxiety is impossible to determine.

Obsessive–compulsive disorder

Imaging studies in obsessive-compulsive disorder (OCD) patients tend to implicate the basal ganglia and inferior frontal lobe in the pathophysiology of the disorder and occasionally of symptom production. Despite the apparent regional specificity, structural imaging studies have had equivocal findings. One study has revealed that OCD patients have reduced volume of the caudate nucleus compared with controls [45]; other studies have indicated increased right caudate volume [46] and a signal intensity asymmetry of the caudate in OCD patients [47]. One of the first fMRI studies in psychiatric disorders was of OCD. Breiter *et al.* [48] observed signal intensity changes in the orbital gyri and dorsolateral prefrontal cortex of OCD patients during symptom provocation.

Studies in OCD, using SPET and PET, have focused on glucose use or regional cerebral blood flow. Although some heterogeneity is found, results indicate differences in metabolic activity and rCBF in the orbitofrontal areas of patients with OCD in addition to findings in the caudate nuclei and the cingulate cortex. As with studies in affective disorders there may be a link with symptomatology. One recent study found decreases in rCBF in the right inferior frontal cortex correlating with illness severity, increased obsessive–compulsive symptoms correlating with a decreased rCBF in the left inferior frontal, medial frontal and right parietal cortex. Furthermore, anxiety and avoidance symptoms correlated with increases in rCBF in the bilateral superior frontal, right inferior frontal, medial frontal cortex and the basal ganglia [49]. Older studies have indicated that the differences in rCBF normalize with an improvement in symptoms [50].

The neuroimaging findings are even more intriguing as they support the neuroanatomical circuitry theory of OCD, which was initially based on the study of patients with demonstrable traumatic brain lesions. This theory postulates that dysfunction of the neuronal circuits linking the frontal lobe with the basal ganglia and other centres is the basis of the formation of obsessions and compulsions [51].

Alcohol and substance abuse

Neuroimaging has a dual role in alcohol and substance abuse, to investigate structural and functional abnormalities that may either be a result or cause of substance abuse.

Chronic alcohol abuse and dependency has been associated with significant cerebral and cerebellar atrophy using CT and MRI techniques [52]. In addition chronic cocaine abusers may have cerebral atrophy on CT scan that correlates both with the degree and duration of abuse [53]. This finding is controversial and is not backed up by more recent MRI studies on poly-drug abusers [54].

Preliminary findings from functional imaging studies using SPET in alcohol abuse have suggested nonspecific regional decreases in cerebral blood flow that correlate with severity of alcoholism and persist after corrections for atrophy. This suggests some neuronal dysfunction independent of neuronal loss [55].

In patients who abuse cocaine, cerebral blood flow studies using SPET and PET have suggested that these patients may have long-term cortical and subcortical perfusion deficits even after abstinence [56, 57]. The study of radiolabelled cocaine with PET has indicated that cocaine is concentrated in the basal ganglia and binds to the dopamine transport mechanism. Use of radiolabelled ligands that bind to the D2 receptor show that chronic cocaine abusers have decreased D2 densities in the striatum that persist through several months of abstinence [58,59].

Studies are currently being conducted using GABA receptor ligands in alcohol abusers and fMRI and MRS in polysubstance abusers. The recent advent of medications for alcohol dependency targeted at the N-methyl-D-aspartate (NMDA) and GABA receptors will provide further impetus for neuroimaging research in substance abuse.

Dementia

A large wealth of research has been conducted to ascertain both the regional and functional significance of cerebral changes in dementia.

Regional cerebral blood flow in Alzheimer's disease, as assessed with PET and SPET, tends to show a reduction in rCBF which, while widespread, tends to be especially marked in the temporal regions, an area especially associated with memory processing. SPET studies using a muscarinic cholinergic receptor ligand have detected focal receptor reductions in acetylcholine receptors in Alzheimer's patients, but once corrected for blood flow abnormalities these are only evident in the most severely affected patients [60]. Additional widespread reductions in receptor densities have been reported in PET studies using a $5HT_2$/D2 receptor ligand [61].

Again the increasing prevalence of dementia within western society and the emergence of effective therapies will make further neuroimaging studies essential, both before and after treatment to correlate with neuropsychological testing.

Conclusion

The brain is the seat of all human emotion and thought and therefore dysfunctions of the brain are the basis of psychiatric disorders. The methods described above have provided an insight into the workings of the intact living human brain. As the sophistication of technology increases exponentially the quality of these research tools will improve. Identified differences in regional cerebral blood flow, metabolism or receptor densities between patient groups and control patients would guide the rational development of new pharmacological approaches to restore these differences to normal. Integration of neuroimaging with other disciplines such as genetics, neuroendocrinology and psychology will allow a greater understanding of the aetiology of mental illness.

References

1. Belliveau JW, Kennedy DN, McKinstry RC, *et al.*: **Functional mapping of the human visual cortex by magnetic resonance imaging.** *Science* 1991, **254**:716–719.

2. Howard R, David A: **Functional MRI for psychiatry.** In *Neurobiology and Psychiatry, vol 3. Neuroimaging.* Edited by Kerwin R, Dawbarn D, McCulloch J, Tamminga C. Cambridge: Cambridge University Press; 1995.

3. Maier M: **In Vivo Magnetic Resonance Spectroscopy, Applications in Psychiatry.** *Br J Psychiatry* 1995, **167**:299–306.

4. Costa DC, Morgan GF, Lassen NA (eds): In *New Trends in Nuclear Neurology and Psychiatry.* John Libby and Co; 1993.

5. Verhoeff NPLG: **Pharmacological implications for neuroreceptor imaging.** *Eur J Nucl Med* 1991, **18**:482– 502.

6. Jarritt PH, Kouris K: **Instrumentation for brain SPET: guidelines and quantification.** In *New Trends in Nuclear Neurology and Psychiatry.* Edited by Costa DC, Morgan GF, Lassen NA. London: John Libbey and Company; 1993.

7. **Talbot PR, Testa HJ: The value of SPET imaging in dementia.** *Nucl Med Commun* 1995, **16**:425–437.

8. Sakas DE, Bullock MR, Patterson J, *et al.*: **Focal cerebral hyperemia after focal head injury in humans: a benign phenomenon?** *J Neurosurg* 1995, **83(suppl 2)**: 277–284.

9. Venz S, Cordes M, Straub HB, *et al.*: **Preoperative evaluation of drug resistant focal epilepsies with ^{123}I- iomazenil SPECT. Comparison with vidio/EEG monitoring and postoperative results.** *Nuklearmedizin* 1994, **33**:189–193.

10. Sawle GV: **Nuclear Medicine and the management of patients with Parkinson's movement disorders.** In *Nuclear Medicine in Clinical Diagnosis and Treatment.* Edited by Murray IPC, Ell PJ. Edinburgh: Churchill Livingstone; 1994.

11. Westera G, Buck A, Burger C, *et al.*: **Carbon-11 and Iodine-123 labelled iomazenil: a direct PET–SPET comparison.** *Eur J Nucl Med* 1996, **23**:5–12.

12. Johnstone EC, Crow TJ, Frith CD, *et al.*: **Cerebral ventricular size and cognitive impairment in chronic schizophrenia.** *Lancet* 1976, **ii**:924–926.

13. Pfefferbaum A, Marsh L: **Structural brain imaging in schizophrenia.** *Clin Neurosci* 1995, **3**:105–111.

14. Pilowsky LS, Kerwin RW, Murray RM: **Schizophrenia: a neurodevelopmental perspective.** *Neuropsychopharmacology* 1993, **9**:83–91.

15. Pettegrew JW, Keshavan MS, Panchalingam K, *et al.*: **Alterations in brain high-energy phosphate and membrane phospholipid metabolism in first-episode, drug-naive schizophrenics. A pilot study of the dorsal prefrontal cortex by in vivo phosphorus 31 nuclear magnetic resonance spectroscopy.** *Arch Gen Psychiatry* 1991, **48**:563–568.

16. Shioiri T, Kato T, Inubushi T, *et al.*: **Correlations of phosphomonoesters measured by phosphorus 31 magnetic resonance spectroscopy in the frontal lobes and negative symptoms in schizophrenia.** *Psychiatry Res* 1994, **55**:223–235.

17. Stanley JA, Williamson PC, Drost DJ, *et al.*: **Membrane phospholipid metabolism and schizophrenia: an *in vivo* 31P MR spectroscopy study.** *Schizophr Res* 1994, **13**: 209–215.

18. Chua SE, McKenna PJ: **Schizophrenia — a Brain Disease? A Critical Review of Structural and Functional Abnormality in the Disorder.** *Br J Psychiatry* 1995, **166**: 563–582.

19. Weinberger DR, Berman KF, Zec RF: **Physiologic dysfunction of dorsolateral prefrontal cortex in schizophrenia I. Regional cerebral blood flow evidence.** *Arch Gen Psychiatry* 1986, 43:114–124.

20. Frith CD, Friston KJ, Herold S, *et al.*: **Regional brain activity in chronic schizophrenic patients during the performance of a verbal fluency task: evidence for failure of inhibition in the left superior temporal cortex.** *Br J Psychiatry* 1995, 167:343–349.

21. Liddle PF, Friston KJ, Frith CD, *et al.*: **Patterns of cerebral blood flow in schizophrenia.** *Br J Psychiatry* 1992, **160**:179–186.

22. Ebmeier KP, Blackwood DHR, Murray C, *et al.*: **Single photon emission tomography with 99m-Tc-exametaz-**

ime in unmedicated schizophrenic patients. *Biological Psychiatry* 1993, **33**:487–495.

23. McGuire PK, Shah GM, Murray RM: **Increased blood flow in Broca's area during auditory hallucinations in schizophrenia.** *Lancet* 1993, **342**:703–706.

24. Selbersweig DA, Stern E, Frith C, *et al.*: **A functional neuroanatomy of hallucinations in schizophrenia.** *Nature* 1995, **378**:176–179.

25. Busatto GF, David AS, Costa DC, *et al.*: **Schizophrenic auditory hallucinations are associated with increased regional cerebral blood flow during verbal memory activation in a study using single photon emission tomography.** *Psychiatry Res* 1995, **61**:255–264.

26. Pilowsky LS, Busatto GF, Taylor M, *et al.*: **Dopamine D_2 receptor occupancy *in vivo* by the novel atypical antipsychotic olanzepine: an 1231-IBZM single photon emission computerised tomography (SPET) study.** *Psychopharmacology* 1996, **124**:148–153.

27. Farde L, Nordstrom AL: **PET analysis indicates atypical central dopamine receptor occupancy in clozapine-treated patients.** *Br J Psychiatry* 1992 (suppl):30–33.

28. Pilowsky LS, Costa DC, Ell PJ, *et al.*: **Clozapine, single photon emission tomography and the D2 dopamine receptor blockade hypothesis of schizophrenia.** *Lancet* 1992, **ii**:199–202.

29. Farde L, Nordstrom AL: **PET examination of central D2 dopamine receptor occupancy in relation to extrapyramidal syndromes in patients being treated with neuroleptic drugs.** *Psychopharmacology Ser* 1992, **10**: 94–100.

30. Busatto GF, Pilowsky LS, Costa DC, *et al.*: **Dopamine D2 receptor blockade in vivo with the novel antipsychotics risperidone and remoxipride—an 123I-IBZM single photon emission tomography (SPET) study.** *Psychopharmacology (Berl)* 1995, **117**:55–61.

31. Woodruff PWR: **Structural Magnetic resonance imaging in psychiatry: the functional psychoses.** In *Neurobiology and Psychiatry, vol 3. NEUROIMAGING.* Edited by Kerwin R, Dawbarn D, McCulloch J, Tamminga C. Cambridge: Cambridge University Press; 1995.

32. Biersack HJ, Klemm E, Grunwald F: **The management of patients with mood disorders, panic disorders and obsessive compulsive diseases.** In *Nuclear Medicine in Clinical Diagnosis and Treatment.* Edited by Murray IPC, Ell PJ. Edinburgh: Churchill Livingstone; 1994.

33. Bench CJ, Frackowiak RS, Dolan RJ: **Changes in regional cerebral blood flow on recovery from depression.** *Psychol Med* 1995, **25**:247–261.

34. D'Haenen H, Bossuyt A, Mertens J, *et al.*: **SPECT Imaging of Serotonin 2 Receptors in Depression.** *Psychiatry Res* 1992, **45**:227–237.

35. Buchsbaum MS, DeLisi LE, Holcomb HH, *et al.*: **Anterior posterior gradients in cerebral glucose use in schizophrenia and affective disorders.** *Arch Gen Psychiatry* 1984, **41**:1159–1166.

36. Buchsbaum MS, Wuh J DeLisi LE *et al.*: **Frontal cortex and basal ganglia metabolic rates assessed by positron emission tomography with (F-18) 2-D-oxyglucose in affective illness.** *J Affect Disord* 1986, **10**:37–152.

37. Bremner JD, Randall P, Scott TM, *et al.*: **MRI-based measurment of hippocampal volume in patients with combat-related posttraumatic stress disorder.** *Am J Psychiatry* 1995, **152**:973–981.

38. Dager SR, Strauss WL, Marro KI, *et al.*: **Proton magnetic resonance spectroscopy investigation of hyperventilation in subjects with panic disorder and comparison subjects.** *Am J Psychiatry* 1995, **152**:666–672.

39. De Cristofaro MTR, Sessarego A, Pupi A, *et al.*: **Brain perfusion abnormalities in drug-naive, lactate-sensitive panic patients: A SPECT study.** *Biological Psychiatry* 1993, **33**:505–512.

40. Rauch SL, Savage CR, Alpert NM, *et al.*: **A positron emission tomographic study of simple phobic provocation.** *Arch Gen Psychiatry* 1995, **52**:20–28.

41. Gur RC, Gur RE, Resnick SM, *et al.*: **The effect of anxiety on cortical cerebral blood flow and metabolism.** *J Cereb Blood Flow Metab* 1987, **1**:173–177.

42. Feistal H, Kaschka WP, Ebert D: **Assessment of cerebral benzodiazepine receptor distribution in anxiety disorders – a study with I-123-Iomazenil.** *J Nucl Med* 1993, **34**(Suppl 5):47P.

43. Schlegal S, Steinert H, Bocklisch A, *et al.*: **Decreased benzodiazepine receptor binding in panic disorder measured by Iomazenil-SPECT. A preliminary report.** *Eur Arch Psychiatry Clinical Neurosci.* 1994, **244**:49–51.

44. Kuikka JT, Pitkanen A, Lepola *et al.*: **Abnormal regional benzodiazepine receptor uptake in the prefrontal cortex in patients with panic disorder.** *Nucl Med Commun* 1995, **16**:273–280.

45. Robinson D, Wu H, Munne RA, *et al.*: **Reduced caudate nucleus volume in obsessive compulsive disorder.** *Arch Gen Psychiatry* 1995, **52**:393–398.

46. Scarone S, Colombo C, Livian S, *et al.*: **Increased right caudate nucleus size in obsessive–compulsive disorder: detection with magnetic resonance imaging.** *Psychiatry* 1992, **45**:115–121.

47. Calabrese G, Colombo C, Bonfanti A, *et al.*: **Caudate nucleus abnormalities in obsessive–compulsive disorder: measurements of MRI signal intensity.** *Psychiatry Res* 1993, **50**:89–92.

48. Breiter HC, Kwong KK, Baker JR *et al.*: **Functional magnetic resonance imaging of symptom provocation in obsessive-compulsive disorder.** Proceedings of the Society of Magnetic Resonance in Medicine, 12th annual meeting, 14–20 August, New York; 1993:58.

49. Lucey JV, Costa DC, Blanes T, *et al.*: **Regional cerebral blood flow in obsessive compulsive disordered patients at rest. Differential correlates with obsessive-compulsive and anxious-avoidant dimensions.** *Br J Psychiatry* 1995, **167**:629–634.

50. Baxter LR, Schwartz JM, Bergman KS, *et al.*: **Caudate glucose metabolic rate changes with both drug and behaviour therapy for Obsessive Compulsive Disorder.** *Arch Gen Psychiatry* 1992, **49**:681–689.

51. Insel TR: **Toward a neuroanatomy of obsessive compulsive disorder.** *Arch Gen Psychiatry* 1992, **49**: 739–744.

52. Hayakawa K, Kumagai H, Suzuki Y, *et al.*: **MR imaging of chronic alcoholism.** *Acta Radiol* 1992, **33**:201–206.

53. Pascual-Leone A, Dhuna A, Anderson DC: **Cerebral atrophy in habitual cocaine abusers: a planimatric CT study.** *Neurology* 1991, **41**:34–38.

54. Liu X, Phillips PL, Resnick SM, *et al.*: **Magnetic resonance imaging reveals no ventriculomegaly in poly drug abusers.** *Acta Neurol Scand* 1995, **92**:83–90.

55. Melgaard B, Henriksen L, Ahlgren P, *et al*: **Regional**

cerebral blood flow in chronic alcoholics measured by single photon emission computerized tomography. *Acta Neurol Scand* 1990, **82**:87–93.

56. Strickland TL, Mena I, Villanueva-Meyer J *et al.*: **Cerebral perfusion and neuropsychological consequences of chronic cocaine abuse.** *J Neuropsychiatry Clin Neurosci* 1993, **5**:419–427.

57. Levin JM, Holman BL, Mendelson JH, *et al.*: **Gender differences in cerebral perfusion in cocaine abuse: technitium-99m-HMPAO SPECT study of drug-abusing women.** *J Nucl Med* 1994, **35**:1902–1909.

58. Volkow ND, Fowler JS, Wolf AP: **Use of positron emission tomography to study cocaine in the human brain.** In *Emerging technologies and new directions in drug abuse research.* Edited by Rapaka RS, Makriyannis A, Kuhar MJ. Rockville:Massachusetts; National Institute on Drug Abuse; 1991:168–179.

59.Volkow ND, Fowler JS, Wolf AP *et al.*: **Effects of chronic cocaine abuse on postsynaptic dopamine receptors.** *Am J Psychiatry* 1990, **147**:719–724.

60. Wyper DJ, Brown D, Patterson J, *et al.*: **Density of acetylcholine receptors in Alzheimer's Disease measured in relation to regional cerebral blood flow.** *J Cereb Blood Flow Metabol* 1993, **13(suppl 1)**:S1.

61. Blin J, Baron JC, Dubois, *et al.*: **Loss of Brain 5-HT$_2$ receptors in Alzheimer's Disease.** *Brain* 1993, **116**: 497–510.

4

Neuroendocrinology

Frances E. Burnett and Timothy G. Dinan

Introduction

An association between disorders of endocrine function and psychiatric, particularly affective, symptoms has long been recognized. A mood state that closely resembles major depressive disorder is a feature of Cushing's syndrome and hypothyroidism, and the mood alteration typically ceases after correction of the endocrine abnormality. Affective change is associated with the administration of exogenous hormones such as glucocorticoids, and thyroid hormones have been used therapeutically as an adjunct to traditional antidepressant therapy.

Peptide hormones released from the hypothalamus to drive the neuroendocrine axes are controlled by the same neurotransmitters that have been implicated in the cause of mood disorders. The limbic system controls mood state as well as sexual and vegetative functions such as sleep and appetite, and has been implicated in the development of psychiatric disorders such as schizophrenia and affective illness. It has close functional links to the hypothalamus, which is the key brain area in the regulation of neuroendocrine function.

Attempts to link endocrine dysfunction with psychiatric disorders have led to an expansion of psychiatric research in the field of neuroendocrinology. The identification of biological trait or state markers of psychiatric disorders would have major implications for psychiatric practice in the areas of diagnosis, treatment and estimation of prognosis. Numerous studies have been performed and various endocrine changes have been linked to psychiatric disorders, in particular depression. In this chapter we review the evidence that links neuroendocrine functional change with depression, schizophrenia and Alzheimer's disease.

The neuroendocrine axes

The neuroendocrine axes are centrally regulated by peptide hormones, or neurohormones, which are released from specialized cells in the hypothalamus (Fig. 4.1). Peptides have complex functions within the central nervous system. Corticotropin releasing hormone (CRH), thyrotropin releasing hormone (TRH) and somatostatin (somatotropin release inhibiting factor) are examples of peptides that function as neurotransmitters and neuromodulators in ways that are quite distinct from their effects on endocrine function.

Peptides involved in neuroendocrine regulation are secreted from cells in the hypothalamus that are stimulated by inputs from central noradrenergic, serotonergic and cholinergic nuclei and that receive inhibitory influences from endogenous opioid- and gamma-aminobutyric acid (GABA)-containing neurones. On release from the hypothalamic cell, the peptide hormone enters the portal hypophyseal blood, which transports it to the anterior lobe of the pituitary gland. There it regulates the release by the anterior pituitary cell of a second generation of hormones into the peripheral circulation to act on the end organ directly or to stimulate the release of a third generation of hormones from the peripheral endocrine organ.

Endocrine function is subject to many regulatory influences in addition to endogenous releasing and inhibiting factors. Most neurohormones are released in a pulsatile fashion, and have a characteristic pattern of release over 24 h known as the circadian rhythm. They are influenced by stress and are subject to inhibitory control by negative feedback, which operates at different levels of the axis.

Several strategies have been used to study endocrine function in relation to psychiatric disorder.

(1) Hormones may be sampled from various sites under basal conditions. Blood, cerebrospinal fluid (CSF), urine and saliva have been analysed for hormone content. This method has several limitations. The effects of circadian rhythm must be taken into account. Most peptide hormones do not cross the blood–brain barrier and may originate from peripheral sources, making serum samples of central nervous system (CNS) neuropeptides difficult to interpret. Peripheral endocrine hormones can, however,

Fig. 4.1 *The neuroendocrine axis. Peptide hormone releasing factors are regulated by a variety of neurotransmitters and neuropeptides. They stimulate the release of secondary hormones from the anterior pituitary cells which enter the systemic circulation to act on the end organ directly. ACTH, adrenocorticotropic hormone; CRH, corticotropin releasing hormone; FSH, follicle stimulating hormone; GH, growth hormone; GHRH, growth hormone releasing hormone; GnRH, gonadotropin releasing hormone; LH, leuteinizing hormone; TRH, thyrotropin releasing hormone; TSH, thyroid stimulating hormone.*

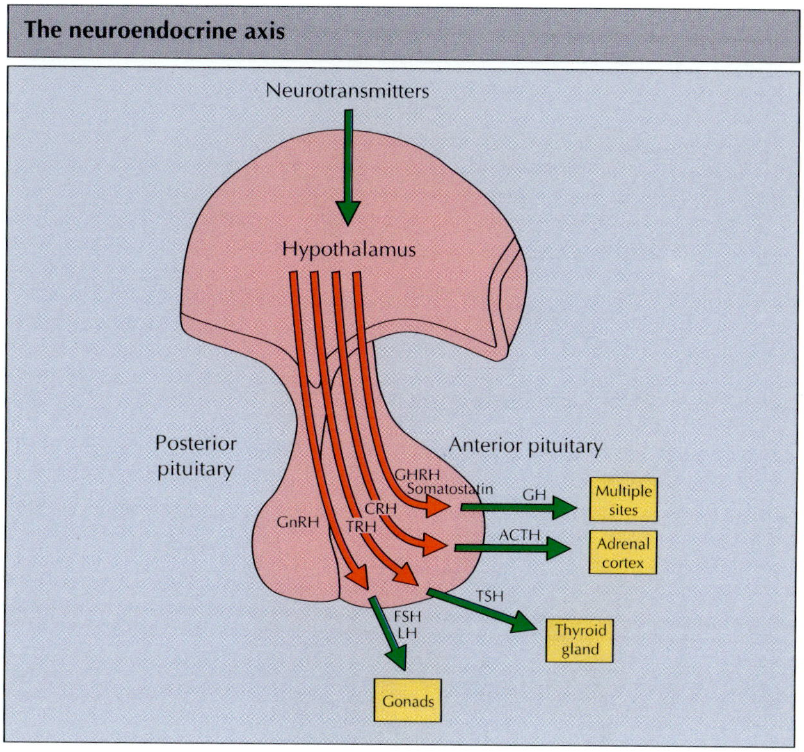

be reliably measured. CSF samples lack information about the source of the peptide, some of which may arise from brain areas outside the neuroendocrine axis or from the spinal cord itself.

(2) Hormones may be sampled over time to detect changes in the pattern of the circadian rhythm. Because circadian rhythms are centrally regulated, loss or change of the characteristic pattern of peaks and troughs may reflect central neuronal dysfunction in psychiatric disorders.

(3) Neuroendocrine function can be tested dynamically using challenge agents, such as exogenously administered releasing factors, e.g. CRH. The dexamethasone suppression test (DST) is an example of a dynamic test that is used to measure the integrity of the adrenocorticotropin (ACTH)–cortisol negative feedback loop. Changes in central neurotransmitter function can be assessed using pharmacological challenge agents, such as the alpha-2 adrenergic agonist clonidine.

Because of the many limitations in using humans, much of the important research has been conducted in other mammals. Chronic stress produces behavioural responses in animals that are an experimental paradigm for depression.

Depression

Links between endocrine dysfunction and psychiatric disorders have been most consistently reported in depression. In this condition, the hypothalamic–pituitary–adrenal (HPA), hypothalamic–pituitary–thyroid (HPT) and hypothalamic–pituitary–growth hormone (HPGH) axes have all been found to be abnormal.

Hypothalamic–pituitary–adrenal axis

In humans, physiological responses to stress are mediated through the HPA axis and the catecholaminergic system (Fig. 4.2). The driving force behind activation of the HPA axis is CRH, which is released from the paraventricular nucleus (PVN) in the hypothalamus into the hypothalamic–hypophyseal portal circulation and transported to the anterior lobe of the pituitary gland. There it stimulates cleavage of pro-opio-melanocortin (POMC), the precursor molecule of ACTH, beta-endorphin and melanocortin. CRH also triggers the release of ACTH from the corticotrope. The effect of CRH is potentiated by arginine vasopressin (AVP), which is released from the same cells in the PVN. Together, CRH and AVP have a powerful synergistic effect on ACTH release.

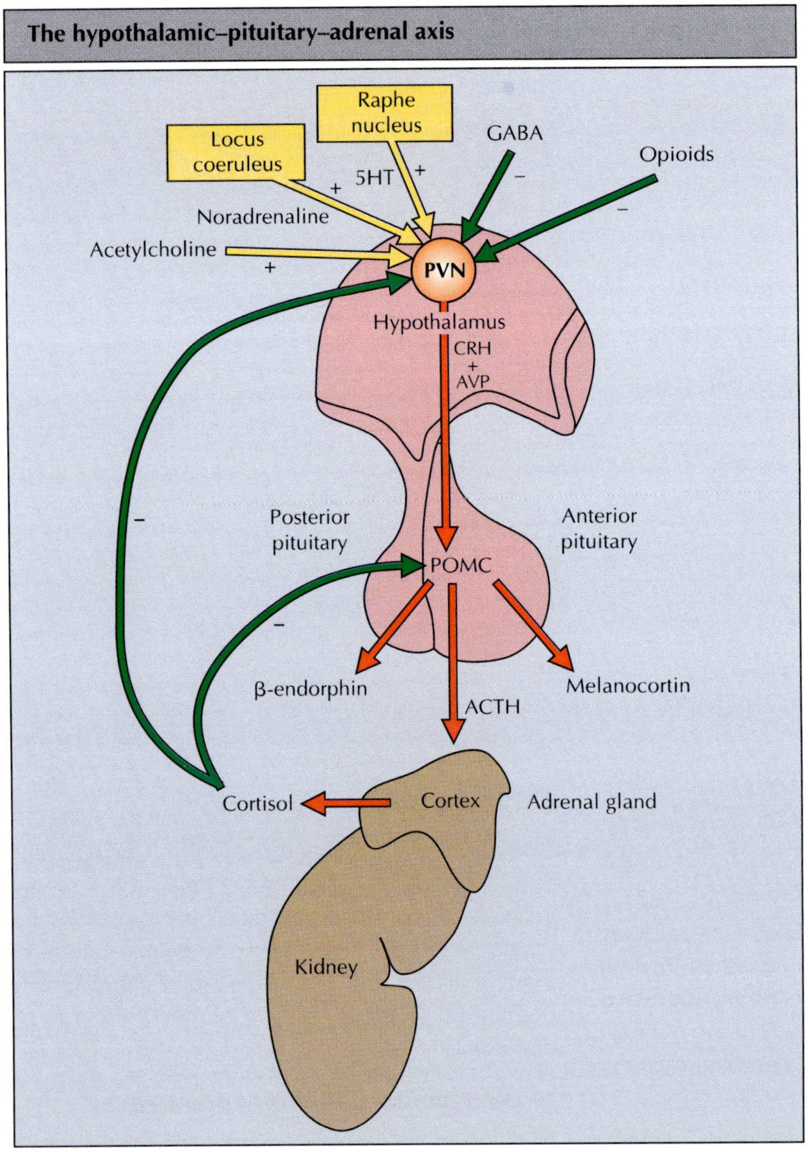

Fig. 4.2 *The hypothalamic–pituitary–adrenal axis. Corticotropin releasing hormone (CRH) and arginine vasopressin (AVP) are released from the parvicellular cells of the paraventricular nucleus (PVN) to stimulate cleavage of pro-opio-melanocortin (POMC) and release of adrenocorticotropic hormone (ACTH) from the corticotrope. Glucocorticoids exert negative feedback to inhibit the axis at pituitary and hypothalamic level. 5HT, serotonin; GABA, gamma-aminobutyric acid.*

ACTH acts peripherally on the adrenal cortex to stimulate production and release of the glucocorticoid cortisol, which has many peripheral effects on metabolic and immune processes. It promotes the redirection of energy by stimulating gluconeogenesis in the liver, inhibiting insulin secretion and stimulating lipolysis. It inhibits immune and inflammatory activity and also induces several enzymes and proteins [1].

Two types of glucocorticoid receptor exist in the brain. The type 1 or mineralocorticoid receptors have a high affinity for cortisol. They are located primarily in the septo-hippocampal complex and are thought to be important in the regulation of circadian rhythm and possibly negative feedback of CRH secretion through hippocampal–hypothalamic pathways. Type 2 or glucocorticoid receptors bind cortisol with much less affinity but are widely distributed in the brain and outside the CNS. They are believed to control negative feedback at the pituitary level and more generally in the axis.

The circadian rhythm of the axis means that the peak of cortisol release is in the early hours of the morning and the trough is in late afternoon or early evening. High concentrations of cortisol induced by stress are inhibited by negative feedback, which operates at pituitary, hypothalamic and hippocampal level. Negative feedback is important in the control of adrenal steroid secretion and in the prevention of the potentially harmful effects of glucocorticoid excess. Three types of feedback have been demonstrated: fast feedback, which is rate-sensitive, acts within seconds or minutes to inhibit ACTH secretion in response to rapidly rising cortisol concentrations irrespective of the steroid concentration. Intermediate feedback is concentration-dependent and reduces ACTH secretion 5–90 min after an increase in circulating adrenal steroid concentrations. Slow feedback acts within hours or days to inhibit expression of POMC messenger RNA (mRNA) and ACTH synthesis in the corticotrope cell, thereby inhibiting both basal and stimulated ACTH secretion [2].

Much evidence indicates that the activity of the HPA axis is increased in depression.

Baseline studies

Hypersecretion of cortisol has been shown in approximately 50% of depressed patients. Urinary free cortisol excretion over 24 h is about twice as high as that in normal individuals. Serum cortisol concentration is also raised, but not to the degree found in Cushing's syndrome, with flattening of the circadian rhythm [3]. Adrenal gland volume is increased by 70% on magnetic resonance imaging [4], and pituitary gland size is also increased compared with normal matched individuals [5]. Evidence that the over-activity of the axis is centrally driven includes the finding of increased amounts of CRH in the CSF of depressed patients and suicide victims [6], and CRH binding sites are reduced in density by 23% in the frontal cortex of suicide victims [7].

Dynamic studies

In normal individuals, negative feedback results in the suppression of cortisol and ACTH production after a loading dose of 1–2 mg dexamethasone. In 50–70% of patients with major depression, cortisol is not suppressed after dexamethasone [8]. An abnormal DST was initially believed to be specific to melancholic depression, and therefore of value as a diagnostic test [9]; however, DST abnormality has subsequently been demonstrated in a range of psychiatric disorders. Non-suppression is found in patients with obsessive–compulsive disorder, panic, dementia, alcohol withdrawal and eating disorders and in normal people who have lost weight. DST non-suppression is present in 4–10% of the normal population.

Nevertheless, severity of depressive symptoms and dexamethasone non-suppression are correlated: almost all depressed patients with psychotic features exhibit dexamethasone non-suppression. As in hypercortisolaemia, the DST usually reverts to normal at or before clinical recovery. Persistently abnormal DST results may have a role in predicting early relapse [10].

Another challenge strategy involves the administration of synthetic ovine CRH. In depression, the rise in ACTH and cortisol is blunted in response to o–CRH stimulation. This could reflect a downregulation of the CRH receptors on the corticotrope in response to chronic CRH hypersecretion and provides further evidence that the overactivity of the HPA axis in depression is centrally driven. Increased CRH secretion could be due to a defect in negative feedback control at or above the level of the hypothalamus or to alterations in monoaminergic or other neuromodulatory systems that exert control over the axis.

Ipsapirone is a $5HT_{1A}$ (serotonin) agonist that results in significantly increased secretion of ACTH and cortisol in humans and rodents. Patients with major depression show blunted responses of HPA axis hormones after ipsapirone challenge, which may reflect reduced function at $5HT_{1A}$ receptors and is consistent with the serotonin hypothesis of depression [11].

The HPA system becomes normal during successful antidepressant treatment [12]. One possible mechanism for this is the ability of antidepressants to alter corticosteroid function. In animals, antidepressants have been shown to increase mineralocorticoid and glucocorticoid receptor density and binding [13], which could lead to enhanced negative feedback. The onset of action of antidepressants on the receptors coincides with their effect on HPA system activity and closely mirrors that of the clinical improvement in depression [13,14]. The primary mechanism of action of antidepressants may be their ability to stimulate corticosteroid receptor function, which leads to correction of the HPA axis abnormalities in depression.

The hypothalamic–pituitary–thyroid system

The HPT system has a similar structure to that of the HPA axis. TRH originates in the hypothalamus and is transported to the anterior pituitary gland in the portal vasculature. It stimulates the synthesis and release of thyroid stimulating hormone (TSH) from the pituitary thyrotrophs into the systemic circulation, where it acts on the thyroid gland causing release of the two principal thyroid hormones, tri-iodothyronine (T3) and thyroxine (T4). Negative feedback operates at the level of the hypothalamus and the anterior pituitary gland. Factors that influence the HPT system include somatostatin and HPA axis hormones, which both have an inhibitory effect.

Dysfunction in the HPT system is frequent in psychiatric patients, particularly those with mood disorders, 20–30% of whom exhibit some abnormality. Mild subclinical hypothyroidism, as detected by a raised basal TSH concentration or an exaggerated response to TRH, is found in many patients with mood disorders, particularly bipolar illness [15]. Antithyroid antibodies have been detected in 20% of depressed patients compared with 5–10% of the normal population [16]. These patients seem to benefit from adjunctive thyroid hormone supplementation.

The TRH stimulation test involves administration of TRH and measurement of the TSH response. Between 20 and 70% of patients with major depression have a blunted TSH response. This blunted response is not, however, specific to depression, as alcoholic patients and some patients with borderline personality may also exhibit a blunted response [3]. Approximately 16% of depressed patients continue to exhibit TSH blunting after clinical recovery. Without information on the premorbid status of these patients, determining whether the abnormality represents a trait marker or is a residual effect from a previous episode of depression is difficult. Residual blunting is associated with an increased risk of relapse [15].

Evidence of hypersecretion of TRH includes increased TRH concentrations in the CSF of depressed patients [17]. Increased TRH secretion results in down-regulation of pituitary TRH receptors, with subsequent blunting of the TSH response. Raised concentrations of cortisol may cause the blunted TSH response in depressive patients. Although some patients exhibit both abnormalities, the two are probably not directly related.

The hypothalamic–pituitary–growth hormone axis

The growth hormone (GH) system is complex, involving many neurotransmitters and hormonal feedback loops (Fig. 4.3). Release of GH from the pituitary somatotrope is controlled by two hypothalamic peptide hormones, growth hormone releasing hormone (GHRH), which is stimulatory, and somatostatin, which is inhibitory. The synthesis of GHRH occurs in the arcuate nucleus of the hypothalamus and is thought to be controlled by the alpha-2 adrenergic system. Somatostatin is released from the hypothalamic periventricular nucleus, where its release is inhibited by acetylcholine [18]. GH is released in a pulsatile fashion over 24 h, with a surge during the first cycle of slow-wave sleep. In the periphery, GH antagonizes insulin directly and other actions such as somatic growth are produced through hepatic manufacture of an insulin-like growth factor (IGF-1), also termed somatomedin-C. IGF-1 inhibits GH secretion at pituitary level and also stimulates somatostatin production in the hypothalamus. Stress, exercise, malnutrition and oestrogens all stimulate GH secretion [19].

Evidence suggests that GH regulation may be abnormal in depression. Frequent sampling of GH during 24 h reveals a change in the pattern of GH secretion, with an apparent increase in daytime secretion, but a reduction in the nocturnal surge. Concentrations of somatostatin in the CSF are reduced in depressed patients but return to normal on clinical recovery.

The insulin tolerance test was the earliest dynamic test to be used in the investigation of depression and the GH response was shown to be blunted. The blunted response may be more dramatic in more severe forms of depressive illness and may persist after clinical recovery. There is a need to control for the adequacy of the hypoglycaemic response, the test is subjectively unpleasant and is no longer widely used.

The most consistently reported abnormality involves challenge with the alpha-2 agonist clonidine. The GH response to stimulation by the drug is blunted in depressive patients, reflecting reduced sensitivity of the postsynaptic alpha-2 adrenergic receptors. Similarly, the GH response to desipramine challenge, also a measure of alpha-2 receptor function, is reduced in depressed patients. These findings may be indicative of more generalized noradrenergic dysfunction in depression. The anticholinesterase pyridostigmine has been found to enhance GH release in depressed patients, compared with controls [20]. This may be secondary to supersensitivity of acetylcholine neurotransmitter function in depression, resulting in diminished somatostatin secretion.

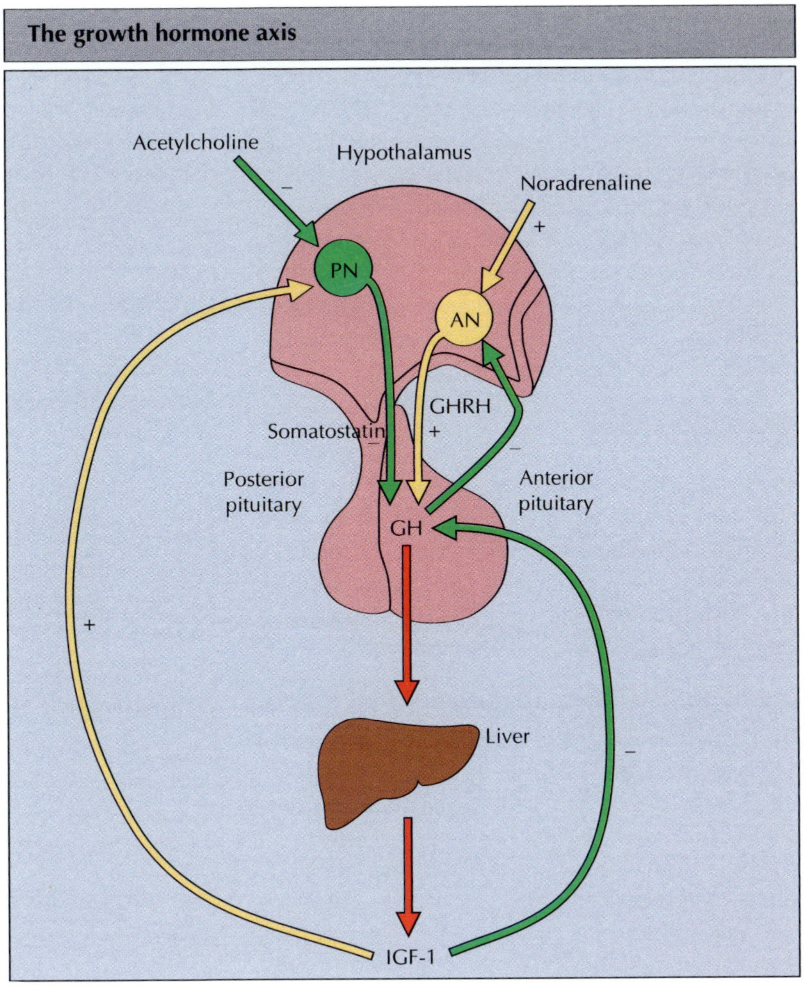

Fig. 4.3 *The growth hormone axis. Growth hormone (GH) secretion from somatrope cells in the anterior pituitary is stimulated by growth hormone releasing hormone (GHRH) from the arcuate nucleus (AN) and inhibited by somatostatin from the periventricular nucleus (PN). Negative feedback control at hypothalamic level means that GH regulates its own production by inhibiting GHRH release, and insulin-like growth factor (IGF-1) has a stimulatory effect on somatostatin production. IGF-1 also exerts an inhibitory effect on GH release at pituitary level.*

Much other work, including challenge with exogenous GHRH, has produced conflicting results. Because the GH system has complex inter-relationships with other endocrine axes, the findings are difficult to interpret. For example, alterations in GH axis function may be secondary to enhanced HPA axis activity. Further research is needed to clarify the role of GH in depression.

Prolactin

Prolactin is released from the lactotroph cells in the anterior pituitary gland. Dopamine has been shown to be the principal prolactin inhibitory factor and TRH, AVP and vasoactive intestinal peptide (VIP) are all thought to be prolactin-releasing factors. Serotonin is known to stimulate prolactin release. Administration of the serotonin precursor L-trytophan causes an increase in prolactin secretion, possibly as a result of an inhibitory effect on dopamine secretion. Intraventricular administration of serotonin in rats causes a decrease in dopamine concentration and an increase in TRH and VIP concentrations in the portal blood. Prolactin, like GH, does not have a specific peripheral target organ but is involved in many physiological processes in many organ systems. The functions of prolactin include the regulation of water and electrolyte balance and control of growth, reproductive actions and metabolic and immune effects [21].

An abnormal prolactin response to various probes has been found in depression. The prolactin response to L-tryptophan has been found to be blunted in depression. D,L-fenfluramine promotes release of serotonin and inhibits its reuptake. In rats and humans, this probe produces a dose-dependent rise in prolactin secretion. Most of the researchers who have measured the response to D-fenfluramine in depressed patients have found it to be blunted.

D-fenfluramine is a more specific probe than the racemic mixture. Its effects on prolactin secretion may be mediated via $5HT_{1A}$, $5HT_2$ and $5HT_{1C}$ receptors. Responses to D-fenfluramine have been shown to be significantly blunted in depressed patients [22]. Clomipramine administered intravenously is a probe for central serotonergic function through the assay of the prolactin response. Blunted prolactin responses are found in depressed patients. These challenge studies produce similar findings and imply that blunted prolactin responses reflect central serotonergic dysfunction in major depression [23].

Schizophrenia

Neuroendocrine mechanisms have been studied much less extensively in schizophrenia. Absence of diagnostic agreement about the core and boundary symptoms and the heterogeneous nature of the illness have caused some difficulties in the interpretation of results of some studies.

The hypothalamic–pituitary–adrenal axis

Examination of HPA axis function has resulted in inconsistent findings. One study showed that acute schizophrenic episodes were associated with dexamethasone non-suppression, whereas studies of chronic schizophrenia suggest that hypercortisolaemia and dexamethasone non-suppression are rare phenomena [24]. Normal ACTH and cortisol responses to CRH have been reported in nine drug-free patients with chronic schizophrenia [25]. So far, the association between functional impairment of the HPA axis and pathophysiology remains unclear.

Growth hormone

GH release is controlled by various monoamines that have been implicated in the pathophysiology of schizophrenia, most notably dopamine, noradrenaline and serotonin. Measurement of basal GH levels in schizophrenia has produced conflicting results; however, nocturnal GH secretion may be reduced [26]. Somatostatin has been found to be reduced in the CSF of patients with schizophrenia and various other psychiatric conditions, suggesting that it may be a non-specific finding [27]. Dynamic studies, using probes, have been performed in an attempt to clarify the picture. In one study, the GH response to GHRH stimulation was not significantly different between schizophrenic patients and control individuals [19]. The release of GH in response to clonidine challenge is used to measure central noradrenergic function. A blunted GH response to clonidine has been observed in some schizophrenic patients but this response may be linked to the presence of affective symptoms [28]. To test both dopaminergic and noradrenergic function, clonidine and apomorphine, a specific D_2 agonist, were given simultaneously to 20 drug-free schizophrenic patients and control patients [29]. Basal concentrations of GH or prolactin did not differ between the two groups. Some patients had a blunted GH response to either clonidine or apomorphine but only two patients had blunted GH responses to both agents. GH responses to pyridostigmine challenge are enhanced in schizophrenia, reflecting possible central cholinergic dysfunction but this may be a non-specific finding [18].

Overall, the scarcity of the data and inconclusive nature of the findings so far make the role of neuroendocrine mechanisms in schizophrenia relatively uncertain.

Alzheimer's disease

It can be difficult to distinguish Alzheimer's disease from other causes of dementia in a living patient. This has prompted the search for a reliable biological marker of the condition.

The cholinergic system

Post-mortem studies have revealed a decrease in the number of cholinergic neurones, and enzymes such as choline acetyl transferase (CAT) and acetylcholinesterase in the brains of patients with Alzheimer's disease. This is widely believed to indicate a central cholinergic deficit. Studies of CSF samples taken from living patients, however, have not shown any consistent abnormality of cholinergic markers. Dynamic studies using the challenge agent physostigmine, a cholinesterase inhibitor, showed blunting of the plasma AVP, beta-endorphin and adrenaline responses, compared with controls. These data suggest decreased responsiveness of the neuroendocrine systems regulated by cholinergic mechanisms in Alzheimer's disease [30].

Studies of endocrine axes

Many patients with Alzheimer's disease have high basal serum cortisol concentrations, and the rate of dexamethasone non-suppression in Alzheimer's disease is similar to that found in depression [31]. Studies attempting to link dexamethasone non-suppression with the rate of cognitive decline have produced inconsistent results [32]. Two groups have reported a blunting of the ACTH response to CRH, consistent with hypersecretion of CRH at the hypothalamic level, but this finding has not been replicated in other studies [33].

In most studies involving the TRH test, blunting of the TSH response is not found [33]. Some patients with Alzheimer's disease have raised concentrations of free T4 in their serum and they have blunted TSH responses, indicating that negative feedback at the pituitary level is intact [33].

Study of the GH axis has relevance to Alzheimer's disease research because of the stimulatory effect of acetylcholine on GH release. Reduced somatostatin concentrations in the CSF and brains of patients with Alzheimer's disease have frequently been reported. Various dynamic tests of the GH axis, using probes such as GHRH and TRH, have produced inconsistent results, undoubtedly reflecting the complexity of the axis [31].

Conclusion

So far, no specific endocrine state or trait markers can be reliably linked with individual psychiatric disorders. The complexity of the relationship between the endocrine axes and central neurotransmitter systems and the diagnostic heterogeneity within psychiatry have further complicated the picture. Certain endocrine abnormalties are, however, associated with specific psychiatric conditions, particularly depression. Whether endocrine abnormalities are of primary aetiological significance or whether they simply reflect central monoaminergic dysfunction remains to be determined.

References

1. Orth DN, Kovacs WJ: **The adrenal cortex.** In *William's Textbook of Endocrinology.* Edited by Wilson JD, Foster DW. Philadelphia: WB Saunders; 1992:486–621.

2. Keller-Wood ME, Dallman MF: **Corticosteroid inhibition of ACTH secretion.** *Endocr Rev* 1984, **5**:1–24.

3. Green AI, Mooney JJ, Posener JA, *et al.*: **Mood disorders: biochemical aspects.** In *Comprehensive Textbook of Psychiatry Vol 6.* Edited by Kaplan HI, Sadock BJ. Baltimore: Williams & Wilkins; 1995:1089–1101.

4. Rubin RT, Phillips JJ, Sadow TF, *et al.*: **Adrenal gland volume in major depression.** *Arch Gen Psychiatry* 1995, **52**:213–218.

5. Krishnan KR, Doraiswamy PM, Lurie SN: **Pituitary size in depression.** *J Clin Endocrinol Metab* 1991, **72**:256– 259.

6. Nemeroff CB, Widerlov E, Bissette G, *et al.*: **Elevated concentrations of CSF corticotropin releasing factor-like immunoreactivity in depressed patients.** *Science* 1984, **226**:1342–1344.

7. Nemeroff CB, Owens MJ, Bissette G, *et al.*: **Reduced corticotropin releasing factor binding sites in the frontal cortex of suicide victims.** *Arch Gen Psychiatry* 1988, **45**:577–579.

8. Stokes PE, Pick GR, Stoll PM, *et al.*: **Pituitary-adrenal function in depressed patients: resistance to dexamethasone suppression.** *J Psychiatr Res* 1975, **12**:271–281.

9. Carroll BJ: **The dexamethasone suppression test for melancholia.** *Br J Psychiatry* 1982, **140**:292–304.

10. Arana GW, Baldesarrini RJ, Ornsteen M: **The dexamethasone suppression test for diagnosis and prognosis in psychiatry.** *Arch Gen Psychiatry* 1985, **42**:1193–1204.

11. Lesch KP, Mayer S, Disselkamp-Tietze J, *et al.*: **$5HT_{1A}$ receptor responsivity in unipolar depression: evaluation of ipsapirone induced ACTH and cortisol secretion in patients and controls.** *Biol Psychiatry* 1990, **28**:620–628.

12. Barden N, Reul JMHM, Holsboer F: **Do antidepressants stabilise mood through actions on the hypo-thalamic-pituitary-adrenocortical system?** *Trends Neurosci* 1995, **18**:6–11.

13. Reul JMHM, Stec I, Soder M, *et al.*: **Chronic treatment of rats with the antidepressant amitriptyline attenuates the activity of the hypothalamic-pituitary-adrenocortical system.** *Endocrinology* 1993, **133**:312– 320.

14. Holsboer F, Leibl R, Hofschuster EJ: **Repeated dexamethasone suppression test during depressive illness. Normalisation of test result compared with clinical improvement.** *J Affect Disord* 1982, **4**:93–101.

15. Holsboer F: **Neuroendocrinology of mood disorders.** In *Psychopharmacology: The Fourth Generation of Progress.* Edited by Bloom FE, Kupfer DJ. New York: Raven Press Ltd; 1995:957–970.

16. Nemeroff CB, Simon JS, Haggerty JJ, *et al.*: **Antithyroid antibodies in depressed patients.** *Am J Psychiatry* 1985, **142**:840–843.

17. Kirkegaard CH, Faber J, Hummer L, *et al.*: **Increased levels of TRH in the cerebrospinal fluid from patients with endogenous depression.** *Psychoneuroendocrinology* 1979, **4**:227–235.

18. O'Keane V, Abel K, Murray RM: **Growth hormone responses to pyridostigmine in schizophrenia.** *Biol Psychiatry* 1994, **36**:582–588.

19. Skare SS, Dysken MW, Billington CJ: **A review of GHRH stimulation test in psychiatry.** *Biol Psychiatry* 1994, **36**:249–265.

20. O'Keane V, O'Flynn K, Lucey JV, *et al.*: **Pyridostigmine-induced growth hormone responses in healthy and depressed subjects: evidence for cholinergic supersensitivity on depression.** *Psychol Med* 1992, **22**: 55–60.

21. Lamberts SW, Macleod RM: **Regulation of prolactin secretion at the level of the lactotroph.** *Physiol Rev* 1990, **70**:279–318.

22. O'Keane V, Dinan TG: **Prolactin and cortisol responses to d-fenfluramine in major depression: evidence for decreased responsivity of central serotonergic function.** *Am J Psychiatry* 1991, **148**:1009–1015.

23. Maes M, Meltzer HY: **The serotonin hypothesis of major depression.** In *Psychopharmacology: The Fourth*

Generation in Progress. Edited by Bloom FE, Kupfer DJ. New York: Raven Press Ltd; 1995:933–944.

24. Holsboer F: **Implications of altered LHPA function for neurobiology of depression.** *Acta Psychiatr Scand* 1988, **341**(suppl):72–111.

25. Roy A, Pickar D, Doran A, *et al.*: **The CRH stimulation test in chronic schizophrenia.** *Am J Psychiatry* 1986, **143**:1393–1397.

26. Kahn RS, Davidson M, Hirschowitz J, *et al.*: **Nocturnal growth hormone secretion in schizophrenic patients and healthy subjects.** *Psychiatry Res* 1991, **41**:155–161.

27. Bissette G, Widerlove E, Walleus H, *et al.*: **Alterations in cerebrospinal fluid concentrations of somatostatin-like immunoreactivity in neuropsychiatric disorders.** *Arch Gen Psychiatry* 1986, **43**:1148–1151.

28. Keks NA, Copolov DL, McKenzie DP, *et al.*: **Growth hormone response to clonidine in neuroleptic-free patients with multidiagnostically defined schizophrenia.** *Psychiatry Res* 1993, **48**:79–90.

29. Brambilla F, Marini S, Saito A, *et al.*: **Noradrenergic and dopaminergic Interrelation in schizophrenia.** *Psychiatry Res* 1994, **53**:231–242.

30. Sunderland T, Molchan SE, Zubenko GS: **Biological markers in alzheimer's disease.** In *Psychopharmacology: The Fourth Generation of Progress.* Edited by Bloom FE, Kupfer DJ. New York: Raven Press Ltd.; 1995:1389–1400.

31. Molchan SE, Hill JL, Mellow AM, *et al.*: **The dexamethasone suppression test in Alzheimer's disease and major depression: relationship to dementia severity, depression and CSF monoamines.** *Int Psychogeriatr* 1990, **2**:99–122.

32. Swanwick GR, Coen RF, Walsh B *et al.*: **The predictive value of HPA axis dysfunction in Alzheimer's disease.** *Biol Psychiatry* 1996, **39**:976–978.

33. Molchan SE, Manji H, Chen G, *et al.*: **The TRH stimulation test in Alzheimers disease and major depression: relationship to clinical and CSF measures.** *Biol Psychiatry* 1991, **30**:567 576.

Schizophrenia

Kathryn Abel

Introduction

Schizophrenia is characterized by adult onset and an incidence of approximately 1% that may be consistent worldwide. Schizophrenia is probably not the result of a single pathological process; increasingly, it is viewed as the clinical manifestation of some aspect of brain disease that may be critically influenced by many non-biological events. Although this chapter is restricted to biological aspects of the disease, different strands of research, such as the epidemiology of environmental risk factors, social outcome studies and the ethnosocial context of the illness are being integrated more and more in an attempt to understand this complex and heterogeneous disorder.

We shall begin with the two most prominent theories of schizophrenia: the genetic and the neurodevelopmental. These inevitably overlap; for example, genetic factors may produce 'neurodevelopmental' defects and vice versa. Neurodevelopmental theories will include aspects of neuropathology from post-mortem and imaging data, and the influence of viral and obstetric insults. We shall also discuss how cognitive neuropsychology is providing new insights into the schizophrenic syndrome and how all of these ideas have been integrated into the theory that schizophrenia is a 'frontotemporal–limbic disconnection' syndrome. In the final section, we shall consider arguably the most heuristic theories of schizophrenia: those concerning possible neurotransmitter abnormalities.

Aetiological theories

Genetic

The concordance rates for monozygotic twins affected by schizophrenia range between 35 and 56%, whereas, for dizygotic twins, the rate falls to about 9–26%. Walker *et al.* [1] suggested that hospital-based studies are biased to produce higher twin concordance rates but they still found about 40% concordance for monozygotic twins from national registers. Adoption studies show that adopted individuals who develop schizophrenia are nearly twice as likely to have a biological parent with schizophrenia than those who do not develop the disorder. These data suggest that schizophrenia is a genetic disease but that less than half of the variance can be explained genetically (Fig. 5.1). In addition, schizophrenia seems to show 'incomplete penetrance', with genetic susceptibility being passed on by an individual who does not express the illness. Gottesman and Bertelsen [3] found that offspring of an unaffected monozygotic twin had the same risk as the offspring of the affected twin. This was not found to be the case for offspring of discordant dizygotic twins.

Owen and McGuffin [4] argue that, even allowing for variable penetrance, schizophrenia is not explicable in terms of a single gene defect. Rather, a form of polygenic inheritance with many interactions with environmental factors is likely. Other factors contributing to the complex genetics of schizophrenia include genetic imprinting and the instability of DNA. Genetic imprinting describes a process whereby genetic material from mothers is expressed differently from that of fathers and may affect the transmission of unstable DNA fragments that can expand from one generation to another. These effects might explain why earlier age at onset and worsening disease severity have been observed in some families.

Most studies of genetic effect have exploited the idea of 'linkage'. This is based on the premise that families with several affected individuals probably 'accumulate' genes of major effect in a heterogeneous disorder. Despite the large number of polymorphic genetic markers, so far in schizophrenia, only one possible susceptibility locus on the short arm of chromosome 6 seems a viable marker and even this is likely to be a small-effect gene. Difficulties with the linkage approach include the instability of results, the possible lack of major gene effects in large pedigrees, the potential difference between schizophrenia from such pedigrees compared with the more usual isolated cases and the inaccuracy of case definition [4]. In addition, linkage is a cross-sectional approach and the varying age-at-onset of the psychoses can mean that studies on the same pedigree at a later date would produce different results.

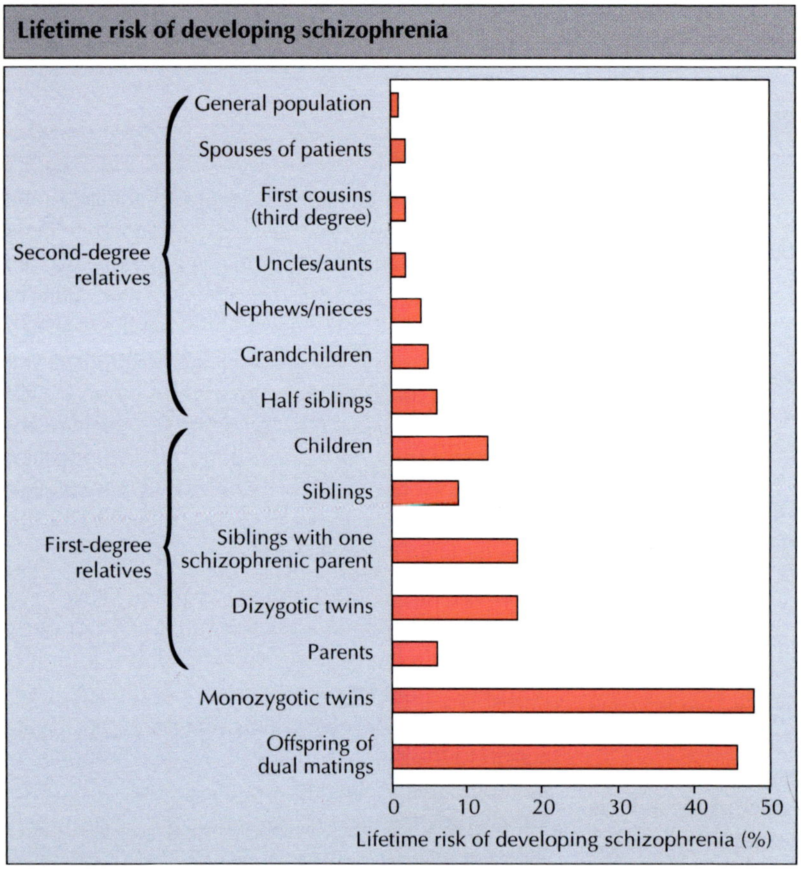

Fig. 5.1 *Lifetime risk of developing schizophrenia. Twin studies of European Populations, 1920–1987. Adapted with permission [2].*

Linkage analysis of allele-sharing in relative pairs goes some way to addressing these issues. Affected relatives inherit identical alleles more frequently than by chance and therefore show allele-sharing despite incomplete penetrance, heterogeneity and multiple phenotypes. This method is further strengthened by a quantitative trait locus (QTL), using dimensions rather than disease categories, so that high schizotypy scores would justify caseness, rather than needing to satisfy criteria for schizophrenia in a relative pair. Finally, 'association' studies compare allele frequencies in groups of affected individuals and a control group. In this way, association is sought between a particular allele and disease presence or absence. To date none of these techniques has produced the positive results hoped for; collaborative studies using allele-sharing, association and QTL techniques offer hope for the future, although a gene effect in schizophrenia will never provide a complete picture.

Neurodevelopmental

Most researchers agree that at least some forms of schizophrenia are neurodevelopmental in origin [5]. This means that an insult occurs to the brain during its development and that this lesion is expressed as poor premorbid social and cognitive functioning during childhood and later in adult life as the symptoms of schizophrenia. Why psychosis only emerges at this stage is not known. Evidence for this notion lies, for the most part, in two areas of research: neuropathological data show abnormalities of neuronal migration in temporal and prefrontal cortex with no scarring or gliotic process, which would indicate a lesion at or around the time of birth. The central nervous system (CNS) develops from three layers of neural tube: the cell-laden ventricular zone, the marginal zone from which afferent fibres develop and the intermediate zone from which the cells in the ventricular layer begin their migration. In mammals, the cortical cellular lamination patterns emerge in an inside-out pattern, with cells destined for superficial layers emerging first. An important aspect of neural development is programmed cell death (PCD); data suggesting abnormalities of these migration processes also suggest that PCD is defective. Such abnormalities of cortical development have been held responsible in part for the abnormalities of frontal-lobe functioning in schizophrenia. Imaging data have corroborated these neuropathological data. Compared with controls, schizophrenic groups show reduced volume of cortical grey matter and temporal lobes and widened ventricular spaces, further pointing to abnormalities of CNS development.

Weinberger [5] suggests that two further strands of evidence are central to the idea that schizophrenia is a neurodevelopmental disorder: lack of progression of the structural abnormalities seen in imaging studies and premorbid deficits, which include cognitive abnormalities and minor physical anomalies (low-set ears, abnormal finger ridge counts and minor neurological deficits), both of which are found in some schizophrenic populations. In a large prospective follow-up study of more than 5000 children [6], investigators found differences between children destined to develop schizophrenia as adults and the general population across a range of developmental domains such as motor milestones, speech and social functioning. They concluded that the origins of schizophrenia may be found in early life.

Viruses

The well documented winter–spring excess of schizophrenic births led to the notion that a viral agent, more prevalent in winter, could produce an intrauterine effect and cause the neurodevelopmental abnormalities proposed above. Maternal influenza has become the most popular candidate for such a viral agent and population-based studies have shown a temporal association between the level of influenza in the environment (e.g. during the 1957–58 epidemic) and the rate of schizophrenia in subsequent birth cohorts that would have been exposed in utero to the influenza virus. However, none of these studies shows a direct association between the mothers who actually developed influenza and the children developing schizophrenia. Sham [7] has argued that, although the data are confusing, the effect seems to be consistent for exposure months 5–7 of gestation (Fig. 5.2). He suggests that, although the effect may be small, the importance of potential influenza-induced maternal autoimmune processes should not be overlooked.

Obstetric complications

Obstetric complications have been associated with the subsequent development of schizophrenia in several studies, although inconsistencies in methodology and the wide range of obstetric events that they encompass often make them difficult to interpret [5]. Furthermore, investigators often had to rely on maternal recall as a method of data collection, which is probably unreliable; studies in which maternal records rather than recall were used as a source of data have generated more consistent results. Given the probability of some association, identifying which specific events are associated with increased risk is important. Prematurity, low birth weight and hypoxia have emerged as important [9]. The effect on rates of schizophrenia, however, is likely to be small.

Cognitive functioning

Intellectual impairment is increasingly accepted as a core feature of schizophrenic illness. Broad neuropsychological testing has revealed that distinguish-

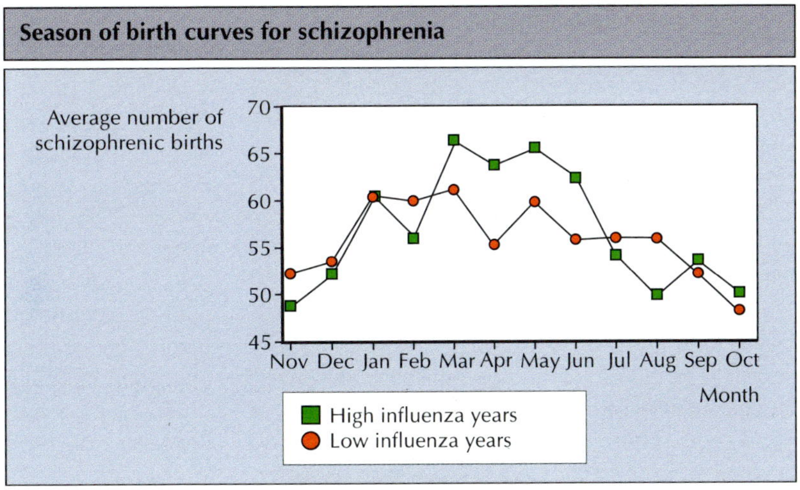

Fig. 5.2 *Season of birth curves for schizophrenia. Average number of births by month during high- and low-influenza years. Adapted with permission [8].*

ing brain-injured patients from those with chronic schizophrenia is difficult [10]. This is less surprising given that our current model of schizophrenia suggests a disease of the brain. Recent research has focused not on whether intellectual impairment occurs, but on the pattern and specificity of that impairment and whether this is a life-long trait or reflects a process of decline during illness from previously normal function. IQ testing and more extensive cognitive batteries have been the mainstay of this research.

IQ testing

In the 1970s, Payne [11] found the mean IQ of more than 100 schizophrenic patients to be in the low average range (96 compared with the normal population average IQ of 100), using the Wechsler Adult Intelligence Scale (WAIS).The catatonic subgroup performed badly, with a mean IQ of 81, compared with the paranoid subgroup, with an average IQ of 95. Whether this deficit was a state or trait phenomenon has been addressed in several recent studies.

Goldberg *et al.* [12] found evidence from scholastic achievement and measures of vocabulary, such as the National Adult Reading Test (NART), that monozygotic twins discordant for schizophrenia performed equally well before illness. After the illness was established in the affected twin, however, consistent discrepancies in cognitive tasks and IQ were found between the discordant pair; whatever the range of function of the affected twin, the non-affected twin performed better. On this basis, Goldberg and Gold [13] comment that '... a simple model in which patients with schizophrenia vary along a severity dimension on cognitive impairment cannot easily be rejected'.

Some investigators believe that the NART may be an inappropriate measure in an illness whose origins stem from early childhood. By contrast, in a prospective cohort study [6], Jones *et al.* found low educational test scores at ages 8,11 and 15 years in children who later developed schizophrenia. David *et al.* [14] identified 195 Swedish army conscripts (out of 50 000 men) who had undergone IQ testing before they developed a schizophrenic illness. These men had recorded IQ scores approximately 5 points less than those of the non-psychotic conscripts. The bulk of evidence implies that schizophrenia is associated with some premorbid deficit of IQ. A consensus exists that many patients who develop schizophrenia have a lower than expected IQ and that this falls further at around the time of their first illness. Whether IQ continues to decline remains a controversial topic [13].

Neurocognitive testing

Batteries of cognitive tests allow broader assessment of cognitive function than simple IQ testing and generally have shown 'across the board' deficits in schizophrenia. Both first-episode, drug-naïve subjects and previously treated patients may have similar patterns of cognitive deficit. Studies of twins have suggested that compared with normal monozygotic twins the non-affected twin of a discordant pair exhibits subtle deficits in, for example, visual and verbal memory, psychomotor speed and scanning and abstraction tasks [15]. A pattern of cognitive deficits affecting memory, motor skills and executive function may be found in schizophrenia. However, attention, language and visual perception may also be affected.

Attention

One of the most consistent findings in both patients and high-risk groups are abnormalities in tests of selective attention and response to specified targets. Examples of this kind of test include the Continuous Performance Test (CPT), reaction time responses, inhibition of the startle reflex, and P50 evoked responses. Typically, patients fail to make use of cues and repeated stimuli, which would normally facilitate responses. In addition, studies have shown that schizophrenic patients are restricted in the amount of information that they can process or use sequentially at any one time [16] and are more distractible than control individuals, finding it difficult to ignore irrelevant stimuli [17].

Language

The clinical description of language in schizophrenia has consistently included restricted expression, such as 'poverty of content of speech' (empty of information, vague or abstract; concrete, repetitive phrasing, poverty of thought). 'Thought disordered' speech, in contrast, includes trains of thought that are illogical, derailed and tangential, such that speech becomes unintelligible. However, on formal testing of expressivity, this group is indistinguishable from normal people. Deficits may occur in the organization of speech and, as a consequence, less flexibility may be found in expression [18]. Little is known about the effects of thought disorder and symptom severity on speech and language; some evidence indicates that neuroleptic treatment improves the logical fluency of schizophrenic speech.

Visual perception

Abnormalities in various aspects of facial perception have been found in several studies in schizophrenia. Archer *et al.* [19] found deficits in facial recognition, facial expression recognition and unfamiliar-face matching tasks. This appears to be distinct from a more simple deficit in emotion recognition [20]. Cutting [21] has proposed that these abnormalities indicate right-hemisphere dysfunction in schizophrenia; paranoid patients may exhibit right-hemisphere facial-recognition deficits, whereas non-paranoid individuals may show left-hemisphere deficits in letter-processing tasks.

Memory

Subtle memory deficits are consistently found in both acute and chronic schizophrenia, which are disproportionate to the overall level of intellectual functioning [22]. Memory abnormalities are seen in verbal learning and recall and in visual tasks [13], although Clare *et al.* [23] found that the rate of learning of procedural tasks (motor-skills) was normal in their chronic schizophrenic group, despite a clear overall decline in performance. Saykin *et al.* [24] suggest that an underlying trait deficit of varying severity may be overlaid with state-related abnormalities, such as those found in performance-related tasks. The trait-related deficits should remain stable over time, whereas the state-related ones may fluctuate with severity of symptoms. Some experts argue that deficits in attention, motivation, effort or information-processing organization can account for these memory abnormalities. However, impairment in recall, recognition, semantic coding and memory and frequency estimation have all been found in schizophrenic groups: these tasks require differences in attentional demand and suggest that attentional deficits cannot account for the memory impairments found. Furthermore, neither psychotic symptoms nor neuroleptic or anticholinergic medication are likely to account for the wide range of subtle deficits seen [25].

Executive function

The Wisconsin Card Sort test (WCST) is a neuropsychological test that is claimed to be sensitive to frontal-lobe functioning or 'executive tasks' (planning, sequencing and initiating plans, monitoring errors with subsequent correction and recovery from any errors made in a given task). This test requires that one use experience to guide behaviour. Schizophrenic or schizotypal patients and first-degree relatives of schizophrenic patients perform consistently poorly on WCST, with deficits of set shifting, response feedback and abstraction and perseverance of errors. The frontal lobe functions to partition and allocate cognitive and memory resources so that complex, novel or dual tasks can be completed and performance on this test may be correlated with social functioning and outcome after hospitalization. Brain-imaging studies have confirmed deficits in frontal-lobe blood flow that correlate with performance impairment on the WCST [26].

Motor function

Motor-performance deficits including failure to adjust to sensory feedback, failure to monitor action execution and perseverance in task performance have all been documented in schizophrenia. Perhaps the best documented motor abnormalities, however, are those of smooth-pursuit eye movements, when patients fail to match the velocity of an object and fail to track objects smoothly [27]. Some evidence indicates that frontal-lobe dysfunction is associated with these specific eye-movement deficits.

Conclusion

Although a global intellectual deficit of IQ is seen in schizophrenic illness, recent research continues to characterize a more focal neuropsychologial disorder that may be specific for schizophrenia. Most investigators believe that neuroleptics improve cognitive functioning in acute illness, although the effect of different agents in chronic stable patients is not well studied.

Frontotemporal–limbic abnormalities

The search for a specific brain abnormality in schizophrenia has been largely unsuccessful. However, recent research has been focused on a possible 'disconnection' in a putative 'frontotemporal–limbic' circuit. On the basis of activation patterns using positron emission data in schizophrenia, Liddle [28] proposed that a subset of patients with schizophrenia exhibited a 'psychomotor poverty syndrome', which shares features seen in patients with frontal-lobe damage, namely poverty of speech, lack of spontaneous movement, social isolation, withdrawal, blunted affect. Neuroimaging also showed decreased activation of regional cerebral blood flow in the dorsolateral prefrontal cortex during the prefrontal executive task of the WCST, which correlated with the degree of such poverty symptoms [5]. A functional 'hypofrontality' was therefore proposed to exist in schizophrenia, which may be linked with symptoms of the psychomotor poverty syndrome.

Focal cellular disease in the frontal lobes of schizophrenic individuals has also led to inferences about cause and function in this disorder. Benes *et al.* [29] found evidence for a loss of tissue or a reduction in the number of small inhibitory interneurones in the superficial layers of prefrontal cortex. Selemon *et al.* [30] found a reduction in the richness of dendritic trees and synaptic connections of the prefrontal area 9 cortical neurones. Neurohistochemistry has also exposed reductions in the amount of nitric oxide synthase containing neurones and a reduction in gene expression for glutamic acid decarboxylase, but no loss of prefrontal neurone numbers [31]. These findings have led to the suggestion that prefrontal cortical development is abnormal in schizophrenia.

Structural neuroimaging has also revealed irregularities in the temporal lobes and limbic areas, including reduction in volume of mesial temporal cortex and of rostral hippocampus [32]. Post-mortem studies, in contrast, point to cytoarchitectural anomalies of entorhinal cortex in layers I and II suggestive of arrested neuronal migration [33]. Weinberger's group have attempted to explain this combination of prefrontal and temporal–limbic abnormalities by suggesting that a lack of integrity in the connectivity between these areas is central to the pathophysiology of schizophrenia. In a study of nine discordant monozygotic twin pairs [34] they found that the more an affected twin differed from an unaffected twin in reduced left hippocampal volume, the more they differed in reduced prefrontal activation during the WCST, measured on regional cerebral blood flow and magnetic resonance imaging. No differences were found in non-affected twin pairs, so this was not a normal relationship between prefrontal function and hippocampal size but only emerged during WCST and with illness. The investigation suggests that, during tasks of working memory such as the WCST, a functional circuit exists coupling temporal and limbic areas (memory and context) and the prefrontal areas (execution of tasks). Hypoactivity may be a consequence of a failure of activation of such a prefrontal–limbic network, which in turn may fail to activate mesolimbic dopaminergic afferents [35].

Neuropharmacology

The monoamines dopamine and serotonin (5HT) and the excitatory amino acid glutamate have all been implicated in a pathophysiological theory of schizophrenia and form the basis of various treatment strategies. Other compounds, such as acetylcholine, noradrenaline and gamma-aminobutyric acid have also been implicated, but provide a less coherent story. These theories depend on the effect of administering to healthy humans drugs that mimic some of the symptoms of schizophrenia (Fig. 5.3). However, none of these drugs adequately mimics schizophrenia and only the N-methyl-D-aspartate (NMDA) receptor antagonists produce the thought disorder so characteristic of this disease.

Dopamine

Twenty years after the introduction of chlorpromazine, the blockade of dopamine D_2 receptors was proposed as the basis of its antipsychotic action. Subsequent potential antipsychotics were judged on their ability to displace dopamine binding agents *in vitro* and clinical efficacy was strictly correlated with potency of dopamine binding (Fig. 5.4). In addition, evidence from postmortem and in-vivo imaging data of increased striatal D2 receptor numbers in schizophrenic patients compared with controls, agreed with notions of subcortical 'hyperdopaminergia'.

In the past decade, however, two events have forced researchers to reappraise concepts of psychosis, antipsychotic drug action and dopamine. First, the discovery of an entire family of novel dopamine receptors, using DNA sequence cloning techniques, taught us that many conventional and unconventional antipsychotic drugs bind to a whole range of dopamine receptors and that the increased numbers of D_2 receptors in areas of human brain may represent subpopulations of D_2-like receptors, such as the D_4 group (Fig. 5.5). Each receptor subtype expresses different qualities: dopamine receptors may activate multiple second messenger pathways; the same receptor may be active in one cell line but not in another; and two receptor subtypes or isoforms may activate the same pathway using different mechanisms. Second, the widespread introduction of the atypical antipsychotic clozapine (particularly efficacious in resistant schizophrenia) has revealed that

Fig. 5.3 *Drugs mimicking schizophrenic symptoms. 5HT, serotonin; NMDA, N-methyl-D-aspartate; PCP, phenylcyclidine.*

Drugs mimicking schizophrenic symptoms

Neurotransmitter represented by drug	Drug	Clinical effect	Schizophrenic-like symptom
Dopamine	Amphetamine Releases and prevents reuptake of dopamine	Excitation, insomnia sensory enhancement, multimodal hallucinations, hyperarousal, hostility, withdrawal	Positive symptoms: hallucinations, mainly visual, tactile delusional mood, paranoia and paranoid delusions
Serotonin	LSD, antagonist and partial agonist at $5HT_{2A}$ and $5HT_{2C}$ receptor; NMDA releases and prevents reuptake of serotonin from synapse	Excitation, insomnia, euphoria, sensory enhancement, mainly visual hallucinations and paranoia, withdrawal	Positive symptoms: dysphoria, mood alteration, ideas of reference, inappropriate affect, concrete thinking
Glutamate	Ketamine and PCP (antagonist at NMDA-receptor)	Anaesthesia, distortions of body image, withdrawal, excitation, delusions, auditory and visual hallucinations, thought disorder	Positive and negative symptoms: negativism, apathy, thought disorder, cognitive deficits

Correlation between neuroleptic D_2 receptor binding affinity and clinical potency

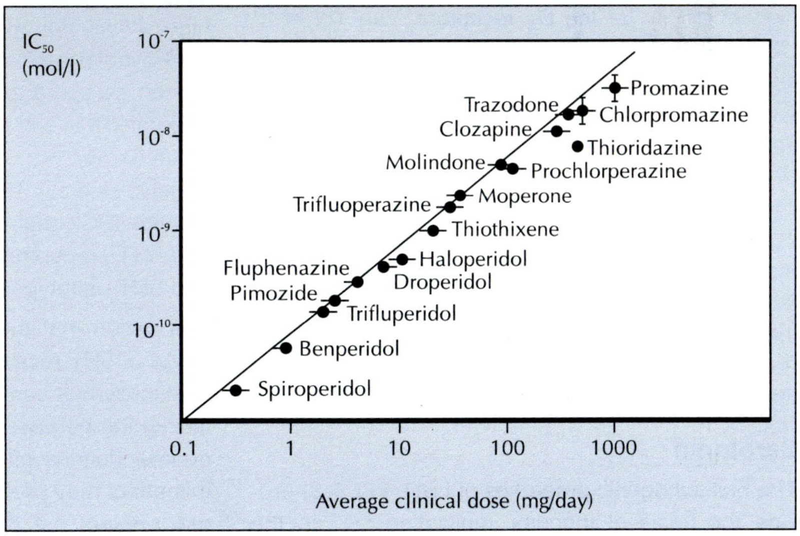

Fig. 5.4 *Correlation between neuroleptic D_2 receptor binding affinity and clinical potency. Adapted with permission [36].*

The dopamine receptor family

	D_1-like		D_2-like		
	D_1	D_5	D_2	D_3	D_4
Distribution	Cortex		Substantia nigra, striatum, limbic	Dentate gyrus, n. accumbens, caudate, putamen	Frontal cortex, dentate gyrus, cerebellum amygdala
cAMP effect	Stimulation	Stimulation	Inhibition	No/small effect	No/small effect
Clozapine affinity constant (Ki[nM])	Modest inhibitor of DA_1 binding *in vitro*		100	200	20
Isoforms	–	–	2 isoforms in $D_{2a;}D_{2b}$	2 isoforms in mice	
Dopamine affinity	+	++	++++	+++	+++
Coexpression of receptors in same neurone	$D_{2,}D_3$	Not known	D_1	D_1	Not known

Fig. 5.5 *The dopamine receptor family. + signifies the relative affinity of dopamine for different receptor subtype.*

D_2 receptor blockade may not be the most important attribute of an antipsychotic drug. Using positron emission tomography (PET) of living brain, Farde *et al.* [37] found that clozapine only occupies 30–60% of D_2 receptors in human striatum, with a higher D occupancy than most conventional drugs; non-responders on classic drugs have higher D_2 occupancy than responders on clozapine. Clozapine also shows highest affinity for the D_4 receptors. Van Tol *et al.* [38] found that the D_4 receptor possessed allelic variants in the population and Sokoloff and Schwartz [39] suggested that these may predict susceptibility to disease states or responsivity to treatment, although Shaikh *et al.* [40] could not confirm this latter prediction and the low-efficacy antipsychotic loxapine has even higher D_4 affinity. Nevertheless, the different profile of dopamine receptor interaction of clozapine and its action at $5HT_2$, muscarinic and alpha receptors has led to alternative hypotheses of schizophrenia, with dopaminergic abnormalities as just one of many possible transmitter anomalies.

Serotonin

The hallucinogenic properties of LSD (Fig. 5.3) provide the basis of theories implicating 5HT in the pathophysiology of schizophrenia. The 5HT model gained some support in the form of post-mortem data showing elevated 5HT concentrations in the basal ganglia, decreased $5HT_2$ receptors in the prefrontal cortex and increased $5HT_2$ and $5HT_{1A}$ receptors in limbic cortices in schizophrenic patients [41]. The greatest impetus, however, has come from the introduction of clozapine, which has high affinity for $5HT_{2A}$ receptors, which are enriched in the medial prefrontal cortex, an area suggested by some to be the focus of neurochemical abnormality in schizophrenia. However, like the dopamine family, the 5HT receptor family is expanding rapidly; at least 14 different receptors have been identified. Clozapine shows high affinity for $5HT_{2C}$ and $5HT_3$ receptors and for the newly cloned $5HT_6$ and $5HT_7$ subtypes.

The notion that the ability of clozapine to block a range of 5HT receptors is central to its antipsychotic efficacy has some compelling data for support: it blocks the behavioural effects of LSD; it blocks the neuroendocrine effects of some 5HT agonists and this effect may predict response to clozapine; and it can prevent the 5HT-induced inhibition of medial prefrontal cell firing, a brain region that may mediate schizophrenic symptoms [41].

In an attempt to identify which aspects of receptor interaction predict atypicality in antipsychotic agents, Roth [42] examined binding affinities for various typical and atypical agents and concluded that potent ratios of $5HT_2$:D_2 binding, $5HT_6$ and $5HT_7$ binding were most likely to predict atypicality. This is consistent with the fact that serotonergic hallucinogens, such as LSD, act via $5HT_{2A}$ or $5HT_{2C}$ receptors and that $5HT_6$ and $5HT_7$ receptors are present in striatal and corticolimbic areas where most antipsychotic drugs act. Measurement of cerebrospinal fluid (CSF) concentrations of dopamine and 5HT, although inconsistent, seems to point to abnormalities in the ratio of CSF dopamine: serotonin metabolites. This again suggests that, with dopamine, 5HT is important in the treatment if not in the pathogenesis of schizophrenia.

Meltzer [43] has proposed a 5HT–dopamine hypothesis of schizophrenia in which he outlines the many different levels at which 5HT influences dopaminergic transmission. This is well illustrated by considering the dense projection of the major serotonergic afferent pathway, the median raphe, which innervates dopamine neurones in the caudate nucleus, cortex, nucleus accumbens and substantia nigra. Meltzer suggests that serotonergic abnormalities may be related to many schizophrenic symptoms in this heterogeneous disorder.

Nearly all new antipsychotic agents exploit serotonergic antagonism with the view that this action may reduce extrapyramidal side effects. This effect may be responsible for the proposed improved efficacy against negative symptoms; however, whether specific 5HT receptor antagonists, such as ketanserin and ritanserin are effective as antipsychotic agents alone remains unclear. Breier [41] proposed that, when depression and extrapyramidal side effects are taken into account, clozapine shows less robust efficacy for negative symptoms; his group have also found that addition of the serotonergic agonist and antidepressant fluoxetine to clozapine-treated patients specifically improved negative symptoms. More specific 5HT-active agents will help to tease out how or whether 5HT affects symptoms in schizophrenia. Some intriguing recent work [44] has suggested that the development of both dopamine and 5HT receptors could be interdependent and that deficits in one neurotransmitter system during critical periods of development could expose alterations in the other system in later life.

Glutamate

Phencyclidine (PCP) binds to a site adjacent to the NMDA receptor of the ubiquitous excitatory neurotransmitter glutamate. In so doing, it non-competitively inhibits the NMDA-mediated effects, such that increasing the amount of glutamate cannot overcome the inhibition. The PCP-induced psychosis model described more than 25 years ago is unique in its mimicry of the schizophrenic state: in submicromolar serum concentrations, PCP can produce exacerbation of schizophrenic symptoms in affected individuals; administered to healthy individuals, it can produce an acute psychosis with hallucinations, bodily distortions and delusions and, in the longer term, features of the negative syndrome, including withdrawal, apathy, disorganization of thought and reversible cognitive changes [45]. Abnormalities of glutamate receptor density and function in schizophrenic brains have also have been reported, although the results are not consistent.

Whereas most models of schizophrenia include dopaminergic dysfunction and all current antipsychotic agents depend on dopaminergic mechanisms, PCP can mimic syndromes typical of dopamine agonists in animals (such as stereotypies and hyperactivity) independent of dopamine [46]. This is probably because glutamate interacts with dopamine *in vivo* in several ways: glutamate may enhance striatal dopamine release via the NMDA receptor; a high potency NMDA-glutamate antagonist (MK108) and a dopamine agonist can act synergistically to produce locomotor activity in dopamine-depleted rats when the individual compounds fail; in the nucleus accumbens, glutamate and dopamine interact to produce inhibitory or excitatory effects, depending on whether D_1 or D_2 receptors are involved [47]. Glutamate may act alone or synergistically or antagonistically with dopamine to produce dopamine-like effects.

Figure 5.6 illustrates how glutamate and dopamine may interact at a subcortical level: the striatum, which has rich D_1 and D_2 dopamine innervation (and ventrally includes the nucleus accumbens) receives cortical, limbic and thalamic excitatory glutamatergic afferents. Striatal activation by glutamate leads to inhibition of the thalamic sensory outflow to the cortex. Cortical afferents release glutamate, which tonically facilitates dopamine release from the striatum, while

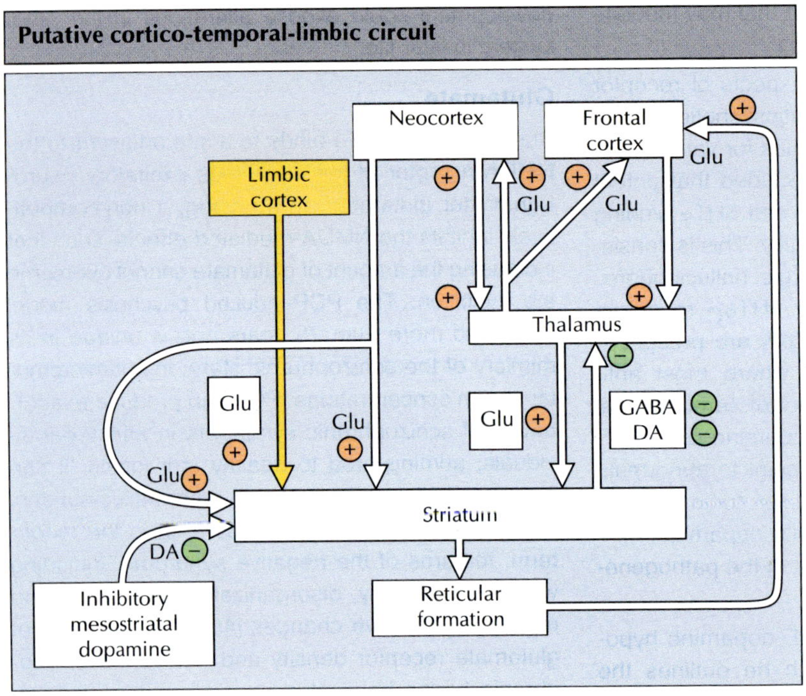

Fig. 5.6 *Putative cortico-temporal-limbic circuit. DA, dopamine; GABA, gamma-aminobutyric acid; Glu, glutamate.*

glutamate release from these afferents is in turn inhibited by dopamine. This negative feedback loop allows the cortex to influence its own sensory input from subcortical structures, such as the thalamus whose output to the cortex is regulated by inhibitory striatal afferents. In this way, the thalamus may act as a kind of sensory filter that limits the amount of information the cortex receives. Bunney *et al.* [48] describe a model to account for the observation that NMDA antagonists (PCP, MK108, ketamine) can both potentiate and inhibit dopaminergic stimulation. They suggest that a direct route from the striatum to the thalamus is under the influence of excitatory nigrostriatal dopamine (via GABAergic interneurones) acting synergistically with cortical glutamate and that an indirect route from the striatum to the thalamus (via GABAergic interneurones) is under inhibitory striatal dopamine control, thus opposing cortical glutamate (Fig. 5.7).

A glutamate hypothesis of schizophrenia holds several therapeutic and aetiological implications. First, other agents such as glycine, polyamines and

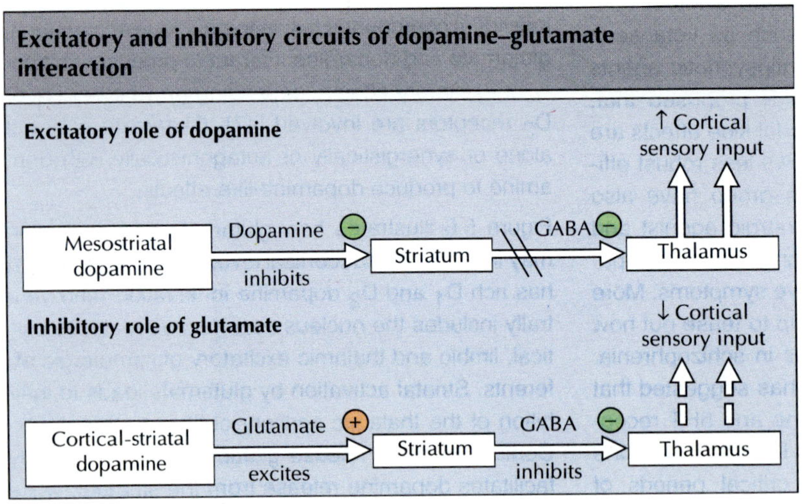

Fig. 5.7 *Excitatory and inhibitory circuits of dopamine–glutamate interaction. GABA, gamma-aminobutyric acid.*

D-cycloserine interact with the NMDA receptor and their therapeutic potential is currently being explored. Second, PCP-like agents can produce cognitive changes similar to those in schizophrenia, but reversibly. Whereas cognitive and neuropsychological changes in schizophrenia had been thought to be core symptoms suggestive of structural or developmental abnormalities that were permanent, the PCP–NMDA effects make this doubtful and open the way for far-reaching therapeutic goals. Third, the psychotic process itself may be neurotoxic, such that hypoglutamatergia or dysfunctional NMDA receptors could lead to hyperdopaminergia and brain damage. Wyatt [49] found that early neuroleptic treatment in first-break psychosis was associated with better outcome and others have cited amphetamine-induced toxicity as similar to that produced by the psychotic process. Despite this, trials of potential therapeutic agents have been disappointing, although a recent study with D-cycloserine added to conventional neuroleptics showed significant benefit [50].

References

1. Walker E, Downey G, Caspi A: **Twin studies of psychopathology: Why do concordance rates vary?** *Schizophr Res* 1991, **5**:211–221.

2. Gottesman II: In *Schizophrenia genesis: the origins of madness.* New Freeman & Co, 1991.

3. Gottesman II, Bertelsen A: **Confirming unexpressed genotypes for schizophrenia. Risks in the offspring of Fischer's Danish identical and fraternal discordant twins.** *Arch Gen Psychiatry* 1989, **46**:867–872.

4. Owen MJ, McGuffin P: **The genetics of schizophrenia: future directions.** *Schizophr Monitor* 1996, **6**:1–5.

5. Weinberger DR: **Neurodevelopmental perspectives on schizophrenia.** In *Psychopharmacology: The Fourth Generation of Progress.* Edited by Bloom FE, Kupfer DJ. New York: Raven Press; 1995.

6. Jones PB, Rodgers B, Murray RM, *et al.*: **Child development risk factors for adult schizophrenia in the British 1946 birth cohort.** *Lancet* 1994, **344**:1398–1402.

7. Sham P: **Schizophrenia and maternal influenza: where we stand now.** *Schizophr Monitor* 1995, **5**:1–5.

8. Sham P, O'Callaghan E, Takei N, *et al.*: **Schizophrenia following prenatal exposure to influenza epidemics between 1939 and 1960.** *Br J Psychiatry* 1992, **160**:461–466.

9. McNeil TF, Cantor-Graae E, Torrey EF, *et al.*: **Obstetric complications in histories of monozygotic twins discordant and concordant for schizophrenia.** *Acta Psychiatrica Scand* 1994, 89:196–204.

10. Malec J: **Neuropsychological assessment of schizophrenia versus brain damage: a review.** *J Nerv Ment Dis* 1978, **166**:507–517.

11. Payne RW: **Cognitive abnormalities.** In *Handbook of Abnormal Psychology.* Edited by Eysenck HJ. London: Pitman; 1973.

12. Goldberg TE, Torrey EF, Berman KB, *et al.*: **Relations between neuropsychological performance and brain morphological and physiological measures in monozygotic twins discordant for schizophrenia: use of an intrapair difference method.** *Psychiatry Res Neuroimag* 1994, **55**:51–61.

13. Goldberg TE, Gold JM: **Neurocognitive functioning in patients with schizophrenia.** In *Psychopharmacology: The Fourth Generation of Progress.* Edited by Bloom FE, Kupfer DJ. New York: Raven Press; 1995.

14. David AS, Malmberg A, Lewis G, *et al.*: **Premorbid neuropsychological performance as a risk factor for schizophrenia: 13-year follow-up of 50 000 conscripts.** *Schizophr Res* 1995, 15:114.

15. Goldberg TE, Torrey EF, Gold JM, *et al.*: **Risk of cognitive impairment in monozygotic twins concordant and discordant for schizophrenia.** *Schizophr Res* 1996, (in press).

16. Asarnow RF, Granholm E, Sherman T: **Span of apprehension in schizophrenia.** In *Handbook of schizophrenia. Vol 5 Neuropsychology, psychophysiology and information processing.* Edited by Steinhauer SR, Gruzelier JH, Zubin J. New York: Elsevier; 1991.

17. Oltmanns TF, Ohayon J, Nezle JM: **The effect of medication and diagnostic criteria on distractibility in schizophrenia.** *J Psychiatr Res* 1979, 14:81–91.

18. Gourovitch M, Goldberg TE, Weinberger DR: **Differential verbal fluency in schizophrenic patients as compared to normal controls.** *Schizophr Res* 1993, **9**: 175–176.

19. Archer J, Hay DC, Young AW: **Face processing in psychiatric conditions.** *Br J Clin Psychology* 1992, **31**: 45–61.

20. Phillips ML, David AS: **Facial processing in schizophrenia and delusional misidentification: cognitive neuropsychiatric approaches.** *Schizophr Res* 1995, **17**: 109–114.

21. Cutting J: *The Right Cerebral Hemisphere and Psychiatric Disorders.* Oxford: Oxford University Press; 1990.

22. Landro NI: **Memory function in schizophrenia.** *Acta Psychiatr Scand* 1994, **90** (suppl 384):87–94.

23. Clare L, McKenna PJ, Mortimer AM, *et al.*: **Memory in schizophrenia: what is impaired and what is preserved?** *Neuropsychologia* 1993, **31**:1225–1241.

24. Saykin AJ, Shtasel DL, Gur RE, *et al.*: **Neuropsychological deficits in neuroleptic naive patients with first-episode schizophrenia.** *Arch Gen Psychiatry* 1994, **51**: 124–131.

25. King DJ: **The effect of neuroleptics on cognitive and psychomotor functioning.** *Br J Psychiatry* 1990, **157**:799–811.

26. Weinberger DR, Berman KF, Chase TN: **Mesocortical dopaminergic function and human cognition.** *Ann NY Acad Sci* 1988, **537**:330–338.

27. Levy DL, Holzman PS, Matthysse S, *et al.*: **Eye tracking dysfunction and schizophrenia: a critical perspective.** *Schiz Bull* 1993, **19**:461–536.

28. Liddle P: **Schizophrenic syndromes, cognitive performance and neurological dysfunction.** *Psychol Med* 1987, **17**:49–57.

29. Benes FM, McSparren J, Bird ED, *et al.*: **Deficits in small interneurons in prefrontal and cingulate cortices of schizophrenic and schizoaffective patients.** *Arch Gen Psychiatry* 1991, **48**:996–1001.

30. Selemon LD, Rajkowska G, Goldman-Rakic P: **Abnormally high neuronal density in the schizophrenic cortex: A morphometric analysis of prefrontal area 9 and occipital area 17.** *Arch Gen Psychiatry* 1995, **52**: 805–818.

31. Akbarian S, Kim JJ, Potkin SG, *et al.*: **Gene expression for glutamic acid decarboxylase is reduced without loss of neurons in prefrontal cortex of schizophrenics.** *Arch Gen Psychiatry* 1995, **52**:258–266.

32. Suddath RL, Christison GW, Torrey EF, *et al.*: **Anatomical abnormalities in the brains of monozygotic twins discordant for schizophrenia.** *N Engl J Med* 1990, **322**: 789–794.

33. Jacob H, Beckman H: **Prenatal developmental disturbances in the limbic disturbances in the limbic allocortex in schizophrenics.** *J Neural Transm* 1986, **65**: 303–326.

34. Weinberger DR, Berman KF, Suddath R *et al.*: **Evidence for dysfuction of a prefrontal-limbic network in schizophrenia: an MRI and rCBF study of discordant monozygotic twins.** *Am J Psychiatry* 1992, **149**:890–897.

35. Weinberger DR: **Anteromedial temporal-prefrontal connectivity: a functional anatomical system implicated in schizophrenia.** In *Psychopathology and the Brain.* Edited by Carroll BJ, Barnett JE. New York: Raven Press; 1991:25–42.

36. Seeman P, Lee T, Chan Wong M, *et al.*: **Antipsychotic drug doses and neuroleptic dopamine receptors.** *Nature* 1976, **261**:717–719.

37. Farde L, Nordstrom AL, Wiesel FA, *et al.*: **Positron emission tomographic analysis of central D_1 and D_2 receptor occupancy in patients treated with classical neuroleptics and clozapine: relation to extrapyramidal side effects.** *Arch Gen Psychiatry* 1992, **49**:538–544.

38. Van Tol HHM, Wu CM, Guan H-G, *et al.*: **Multiple dopamine D_4 receptor variants in the human population.** *Nature* 1992, **358**:149–152.

39. Sokoloff P, Schwartz J-C: **Novel dopamine receptors half a decade later.** *Trends Pharmacol Sci* 1995, **16**:270–275.

40. Shaikh S, Collier D, Kerwin RW, *et al.*: **Dopamine D_4 receptor subtypes and response to clozapine.** *Lancet* 1993, **341**:116.

41. Breier A: **Serotonin, schizophrenia and antipsychotic drug action.** *Schiz Res* 1995, **14**:187–202.

42. Roth BL: **Atypical antipsychotic drugs: Which receptors are relevant?** *Proceedings of IBC conference: Serotonin receptors in the Central Nervous System.* Philadelphia: Jan 25–26.

43. Meltzer HY: **Clinical studies in the mechanism of action of clozapine: the dopamine–serotonin hypothesis of schizophrenia.** *Psychopharmacology* 1989, **99**: 518–527.

44. Roth BL, Meltzer HY: **The role of serotonin in schizophrenia.** In *Psychopharmacology: A Fourth Generation in Progress, chapter 102.* Edited by Bloom FE, Kupfer DJ. New York: Raven Press;1995: 1215–1228.

45. Javitt DC, Zutkin SR: **Recent advances In phenylcyclidine model of schizophrenia.** *Am J Psychiatry* 1991, **148**:1301–1308.

46. Carlsson M, Carlsson A: **Schizophrenia: A subcortical neurotransmitter imbalance syndrome?** *Schizophr Bull* 1990, **16**:425–432.

47. Svensson A, Carlsson ML, Carlsson A: **Interaction between glutamatergic and dopaminergic tone in the nucleus accumbens of mice. Evidence of a dual glutamatergic function with respect to psychomotor control.** *J Neural Transm* 1992, **88**:235–240.

48. Bunney BG, Bunney WE, Carlsson A: **Schizophrenia and glutamate.** In *Psychopharmacology: The Fourth Generation of Progress.* Edited by Bloom FE, Kupfer DJ. New York: Raven Press; 1995:1205–1214.

49. Wyatt RJ: **Neuroleptics and the natural course of schizophrenia.** *Schizophr Bull* 1991, **17**:325–351.

50. Goff DC, Tsai G, Mananoch DS, *et al.*: **Dose finding trial for D-cycloserine added to neuroleptics for negative symptoms in schizophrenia.** *Am J Psychiatry* 1995, **152**:1213–1215.

Mood disorders

Jogin H. Thakore

Introduction

The term 'mood disorders' covers various conditions, including depressive disorders and bipolar affective disorder, linked together by a group of symptoms relating to mood, behaviour and cognition. Depressive disorders include the subtypes of major depressive disorder (melancholic, atypical, catatonic) and dysthymic disorder. Dysthymic disorder refers to an illness of low-grade chronicity (2 years), with insidious onset and an intermittent or persistent course which has usually started in adolescence or childhood.

Affective disorders incorporate quite diverse phenomenological conditions. Some differences between the various subsets of these disorders have been recorded in large multicentre trials conducted in the USA.

Bipolar disorder: one or more manic episodes (bipolar I) with or without a major depressive episode and a major depressive disorder with hypomanic episodes (bipolar II)

Cyclothymia: mood swings that fail to meet the criteria for a bipolar I or bipolar II disorder

Rapid cycling disorder: four or more affective episodes in 1 year

Epidemiology

The lifetime prevalence of unipolar depression is 12% for women and 8% for men; although men are more likely to commit suicide [1]. The rates of unipolar depression are rising and various hypotheses have been formulated to try to explain this worrying trend. These range from depression being more frequently diagnosed in younger people, to higher rates of chronicity and lack of compliance with treatment. Surveying both institutionalized and community groups in five different centres involving over 18 000 people across the USA, the Epidemiological Catchment Area [2] study revealed that people aged less than 45 years had the highest rates of all mood disorders. No difference was seen between the sexes in the prevalence of bipolar affective disorder, although women were more likely to suffer from unipolar depression and dysthymia. The incidence of mood disorders is approximately 1.59%. Only half of those with bipolar I disorder and major depressive illness recover within 1 year and less than 30% go into remission during the next 5 years. Not only do mood disorders occur frequently in the general population, but they are associated with a potentially debilitating chronicity. Little doubt exists that biological factors play a major part in the pathogenesis of mood disorders.

Major biological theories

Genetic theories

Genetic epidemiology has relied on four methods by which to study the familial basis of affective disorders (Fig. 6.1).

Genetic epidemiology

Study	Measure
Family	The aggregation of an illness in the family of affected individual
Twin	The comparison of the concordance rates between monozygotic and dizygotic twins
Adoption	The differential rates of illness expression between the biological and adoptive parents of probands
Genetic	Associations between known genetic traits and illnesses, either within families or across families

Fig. 6.1 *Genetic epidemiology.*

Family studies

A review of family studies conducted in mood disorders [3] found that only four reports for bipolar and five for unipolar depression fulfilled strict methodological criteria which allowed a reasonable interpretation of their results. The absolute risk of depression was increased approximately twofold for both types of disorder and some degree of specificity of transmission was found in that the two types of conditions tend to breed true.

Twin studies

A fivefold difference in the concordance rates of bipolar depression between monozygotic twins (60%) and dizygotic twins (12%) has long been observed [4]. In contrast, a modest difference is seen in the concordance rates of unipolar depression between the two types of twins (a 1.2–1.9-fold increase in monozygotic twins) [5,6]. The application of quantitative models, however, indicates that the variance due to genetic factors plays a significant part in the pathogenesis of major depressive illness.

Adoption studies

Three major adoption studies have been carried out: two were positive in their findings whereas the third was not [7–9]. The rates of depression in the positive studies were increased 15-fold in the natural parents of the affected adoptees compared with their foster parents.

Genetic marker studies

Association studies

A trait, in order to be a biological marker must fulfil the following criteria:

- be associated with an increased risk of illness
- be present during the recovery and active phases of an illness
- be independent of the disease

Numerous studies have examined the relationship between mood disorders and blood groups (ABO), human leucocyte antigens and monoamine oxidase. Low monoamine oxidase activity has been found in a number of psychiatric illnesses and appears to reflect non-specific alteration in other neurochemical systems. A recent study [10] using molecular biological techniques has shown a possible association between bipolar I disorder and monoamine oxidase activity.

Linkage studies

Recombination, an exchange of segments between chromosomes, occurs during meiosis when pairs of homologous chromosomes come together. The farther apart two genes are from each other, the more likely they are to undergo recombination. In linkage analysis the co-inheritance of the marker and the disease gene are followed within a family. Two major methods of linkage analysis are the sib-pair method and logarithm of odds (Lod) score method. The sib-pair method looks at the co-occurrence of marker alleles at a locus among affected sibling pairs. No firm evidence exists for a linkage between human leucocyte antigen markers and mood disorders; two studies have shown a link while eight have not.

The Lod score is a ratio that calculates the odds for (and against) the degree of linkage. A Lod score of more than 3 implies that the odds that the two loci are linked by mere chance alone are 1000:1. A review of three articles [11] illustrates the use of the Lod score method in bipolar depression. One study looked for alleles that were inherited more often than by chance on chromosomes 6, 13 and 15 and generated an Lod score of 1.5–2.0. Critics of the study have claimed that a Lod score of 1.5–2.0 merely reflects background noise. Linkage disequilibrium, studied in another trial found a mutation on the long arm of chromosome 18: in people with mental disorders extended chromosomal regions are inherited with disease genes more often than in controls. Certain disease-causing dominant genes have also been pinpointed using traditional linkage analysis methods. Although these results are exciting, no firm conclusions can be made until they have been replicated.

Psychoneuroimmunology

The immune system is capable of discriminating 'self' from 'non-self' thereby affording protection from various antigens (foreign substances). The immune system comprises three working groups of cells: T cells, B cells, and natural killer cells. Humoral responses are mediated by B cells and their products while cellular responses are mediated by T cells. The two types of cells interact to produce the immune response. Natural killer cells differ from the other two cell types in that they are immunologically 'non-specific' and do not require sensitization to specific antigens before they display cytotoxic activity. The immune system can be evaluated by cell counts or counts of cell subsets and by determining the functional capability of cellular and humoral responses.

Major depression is associated with moderate leucocytosis, higher antibody titres (for example, antiphospholipid), alterations in the levels and ratios of various T-cell subsets, B-cell proliferation, higher production rates of interleukin-1 and interleukin-6 and higher concentrations of acute phase protein responses [12]. Reviews of the psychoneuroimmune aspects of major depression have reported that results are 'inconclusive and inconsistent' [13], 'lowered measures of immunocompetence' [14], and 'lowered measure of all immune functions' [15]. The discrepancies between the studies are methodological: variables such as age, gender and severity of symptoms were not taken into account. Future investigators need to allow for such factors and also report on the specificity of these immune disturbances in conditions other than major depression.

Neuroimaging findings

Diagnostic radiology has provided two major types of investigative paradigms for research in mood disorders. Structural findings have helped elucidate the neuroanatomical basis of these illnesses while functional studies, primarily employing single photon emission computed tomography (SPECT) and positron emission tomography (PET), have proved a useful means by which to study cerebral blood flow and cerebral metabolic rate.

Structural changes

Computed tomography and magnetic resonance imaging have shown few consistent findings in mood disorders, compared with those found in schizophrenia. The most frequently reported finding is an increased ventricle to brain ratio, in particular enlargement of the lateral ventricles. A meta-analysis of studies [16] examining sulcal and ventricular enlargement or both concluded that mood disorders are associated with such abnormalities but less so than schizophrenia.

Abnormalities have also been found in the white matter of young- and old-onset patients with both unipolar and bipolar depression. Hyperintensities have been located in the basal ganglia and subcortical tissue including the thalamus and pons. One review [17] has shown an association between white matter lesions and cognitive impairment in patients with bipolar disorders. These changes are non-specific, however, and their significance is unknown.

A series of studies using computed tomography and magnetic resonance imaging has examined the hypothalamic–pituitary–adrenal axis in patients with mood disorders. One study [18] has shown a relationship between hippocampal volume (the hippocampus contains a large number of steroid receptors that are involved in 'switching off' the hypothalamic–pituitary–adrenal axis) and cortisol levels at 23:00 h. No differences were seen in hippocampal size between depressive patients and controls. Unipolar depressive patients [19] had large pituitaries in one study, while another [20] showed a positive relationship between pituitary volume and post-dexamethasone cortisol levels. The decrease in adrenal gland volume seen with antidepressant exposure in depressive patients indicates that enlarged adrenals are a state-dependent phenomenon [21].

Functional changes

PET and SPECT scan studies in mood disorders have shown that even though hypometabolism occurs globally it is particularly prominent in the frontal and temporal lobes. This abnormality may be state-dependent as it improves with treatment. Activation studies, which involve the patient giving their attention to a predetermined task, reveal that abnormal activation occurs in the frontal and temporal lobes, amygdala and cingulate cortex.

Recent SPECT scan studies [22] in unipolar depression have revealed a bilateral increase in ^{99m}Tc-exametazime uptake in the inferior anterior cingulate cortex and thalamus both before and after treatment, whereas another study [23] found paralimbic hypoperfusion. One PET scan study [24] found an overall decrease in type-2 dopaminergic receptors in the brains of unipolar depressive patients whereas another [25] showed blunted regional glucose metabolism responses to the racemic mixture of fenfluramine [a potent releaser of 5-hydroxytryptamine (5-HT; serotonin). These studies represent important steps in confirming the indoleamine hypothesis of affective disorders.

Biochemical theories

The catecholaminergic theory of affective disorders, stating that depression was associated with a deficit of noradrenergic neurotransmission, was first published by Schildkraut in 1965 [26]. The concept was later expanded to include an abnormality of serotonergic function [27]. Such hypotheses were based on three assumptions:

- Reserpine, an antihypertensive with the ability to release and deplete catecholaminergic stores, was capable of inducing depression.
- Reserpine when given to rats produced a behavioural picture that was believed to mimic depression.
- Imipramine, the tricyclic antidepressant introduced in 1957, acted by inhibiting the reuptake of noradrenaline and 5HT and was effective in treating depression.

This rather simplistic view of a synaptic abnormality of catecholaminergic transmission has been challenged, however, by many observations. Although clinical remission may take up to 2–6 weeks, synaptic deficits are corrected within 24 h of being exposed to an antidepressant. Furthermore, not all effective antidepressants are monoamine reuptake inhibitors, for example, mianserin is believed to act as an alpha-2 adrenergic antagonist (alpha-2 adrenergic presynaptic autoreceptors are responsible for decreasing secretion of monoamines).

Modern versions of the monoamine theory of depression, address monoamine activity and receptor/second messenger abnormalities [28,29]. Evidence of a dysfunctional noradrenergic system comes from a variety of sources. Plasma and urinary measurements of 3-methoxy-4-hydroxy phenyl glycol (MHPG) (the primary metabolite of noradrenaline) are consistently lower in bipolar and unipolar depressive patients than in controls. In fact, low MHPG levels predict a good response to tricyclic antidepressants. Surprisingly, plasma and urinary concentrations of noradrenaline and adrenaline are elevated in bipolar and unipolar depressive patients suggesting an increased turnover of catecholamines from an overactive sympathetic nervous system. Manic episodes are typically associated with increased catecholaminergic activity, although to a higher degree than the depressive phase of bipolar illness or indeed in unipolar depression. Lithium treatment results in a decrease of sympathetic nervous system activity in both responders and non-responders, indicating that this decrease is a necessary but not an absolute prerequisite for remission.

Longitudinal studies looking at the effects of antidepressant treatment with either tricyclics or selective serotonin reuptake inhibitors on catecholaminergic turnover show that the latter decrease with time. This decrease, however, occurs in both treatment responders and non-responders. Lastly, many studies have found a positive relationship between indicators of noradrenergic function and hypothalamic–pituitary–adrenal axis. The significance of this association is as yet unknown and may reflect a 'stress'-induced stimulation of both the hypothalamic–pituitary–adrenal axis and the sympathetic nervous system or a corticotropin-releasing hormone-induced activation of both systems.

Abnormalities of both alpha- and beta-adrenergic receptors and their second messenger systems have been implicated in depression. Platelet aggregation is normally mediated by alpha-2-adrenergic receptors and adrenaline suppresses platelet adenylate cyclase activity. Depressive patients have increased alpha-2-adrenergic-induced platelet aggregation and blunted adenylate cyclase responses to clonidine, an alpha-2-adrenergic agonist. Stimulation of alpha-2-adrenergic receptors by clonidine results in the release of growth hormone-releasing hormone and subsequently growth hormone in normal volunteers. Blunted clonidine-induced growth hormone responses are seen in depressive patients indicating subsensitive alpha-2-adrenergic receptors.

Beta-adrenergic receptors number have decreased in rats following chronic treatment with antidepressants. Increased beta-adrenergic receptor activity has been observed by some but not all, in the cortices of patients who have committed suicide. In contrast, the lymphocytes of depressive patients have lower numbers of beta-adrenergic receptors than controls and are far less sensitive to activation with various beta-adrenergic agonists. This change in lymphocyte activity may represent a compensatory mechanism for an overactive sympathetic nervous system.

As mentioned earlier, a decrease in serotonergic function has been implicated in the pathogenesis of major depression. Deficits in 5HT activity may represent an important cause of depression or merely indicate a propensity to become depressed; various studies have supported this hypothesis. L-tryptophan is the precursor to 5HT and its plasma concentrations or the ratio of L-tryptophan to the sum of competing amino acids (this ratio provides a measure of the amount of L-tryptophan available to the brain) has been found to be reduced in major depression. In fact, a negative association is seen between this ratio and response to antidepressant treatment.

Platelets are considered to be a model for central 5HT neurones as both neurones and platelets are capable of taking up, storing and releasing 5HT. The rate of uptake of 5HT has been shown to be reduced in patients with depression. Lower numbers of [^{3}H]imipramine binding sites are found on platelets from depressive patients; however, these sites are heterogeneous (they exist in high and low affinity forms). [^{3}H]Paroxetine binds to the 5HT transporter with much greater specificity although to date, differences between controls and patients with depression have been inconsistent.

Cerebrospinal fluid levels of 5-hydroxyindoleacetic acid (5HIAA) and post-mortem tissue concentrations of 5HT receptors and 5HIAA are indirect measures of central serotonergic activity. Some studies have reported lower levels of 5HIAA in the cerebrospinal fluid and neuronal tissue of patients who have committed suicide, this has not been replicated in other studies. Low cerebrospinal fluid 5HIAA levels are indicative of higher suicide risk rather than depression.

Molecular biology and pharmacological probes have identified a number of different serotonergic receptors. Postsynaptic $5HT_2$ receptors are located centrally in the cortex, and peripherally on platelets. $5HT_2$ binding and second messenger system activity have been shown to be increased on the platelets of patients with major depression. In normal volunteers, slow wave sleep increases in response to blocking $5HT_2$ receptors with antagonists such as ritanserin or cyproheptadine. No such increase is observed in depression, providing further evidence of $5HT_2$ receptor dysfunction. In depression, levels of frontal cortex $5HT_2$ receptors have increased or been no different to levels in normal volunteers. Levels of $5HT_1$ receptors have been found to be increased in the prefrontal cortices, although decreased in the amygdala and hippocampus of depressed patients who have committed suicide. Whether these abnormalities are the 'root cause' of mood disorders is as yet unknown; however, these disorders are characterized by dysfunctional serotonergic and noradrenergic systems.

Conclusion

Despite the large amount of literature on the biological basis of mood disorders, no biological markers unique for either type of affective disorder have been discovered. Until a highly specific method of identifying these illnesses becomes available, most investigations are probably being performed on a heterogeneous group of subjects. This may well explain the discrepancies observed in research conducted within mood disorders.

References

1. Andreasen NC, Scheftner W, Reich T, *et al.*: **The validation of the concept of endogenous depression: a family study approach.** *Arch Gen Psychiatry* 1986, **43**: 246–251.

2. Robins LN, Helzer JE, Weissman MM, *et al.*: **Lifetime prevalence of specific psychiatric disorder in three sites.** *Arch Gen Psychiatry* 1985, **41**:949–958.

3. Taylor MA, Berenbaum SA, Jampala VC, *et al.*: **Are schizophrenia and affective disorders related? Preliminary data from a family study.** *Am J Psychiatry* 1993, **150**:278–285.

4. Bertelsen A, Harvald B, Hauge M: **A Danish twin study of manic-depressive disorders.** *Br J Psychiatry* 1977, **130**:330–351.

5. Kendler KS, Neale M, C, Kessler RC, *et al.*: **A population-based twin study of major depression in women: the impact of varying definitions of illness.** *Arch Gen Psychiatry* 1992, **49**:257–267.

6. McGuffin P, Katz R: **The genetics of manic-depressive disorder.** *Br J Psychiatry* 1989, **155**:294–304.

7. Mendlewicz J, Rainer JD: **Adoption study supporting genetic transmission in manic-depressive illness.** *Nature* 1977, 268:327–329.

8. Wender PH, Kety SS, Rosenthal D, *et al.*: **Psychiatric disorders in the biological and adoptive families and adopted individuals with affective disorders.** *Arch Gen Psychiatry* 1986, **43**:923–929.

9. Cadoret RJ, O'Gorman TW, Heywood E *et al.*: **Genetic and environmental factors in major depression.** *J Affect Disord* 1985, **9**:155–164.

10. Mendlewicz J, Sevy S, Mendlebaum K: **Molecular genetics in affective illness [Mini-review].** *Life Sci* 1993, **52**: 231–242.

11. Morrell V: **Manic depressive findings spark polarised debate.** *Science* 1996, **272**:31–32.

12. Maes M, Meltzer HY, Stevens W, *et al.*: **Multiple reciprocal relationships between in vivo cellular immunity hypothalamic-pituitary-adrenal axis in depression.** *Psychol Med* 1994, **24**:167–177.

13. Stein M, Miller AH, Trestman RL: **Depression, the immune system, health and illness.** *Arch Gen Psychiatry* 1991, **48**:171–177.

14. Herbert TB, Cohen S: **Stress and immunity: a meta-analytic review.** *Psychosom Med* 1993, **55**:364–379.

15. Weisse CS: **Depression and immunocompetence: a review of the literature.** *Psychol Bull* 1992, **111**:475–489.

16. Elkis H, Friedman L, Wise A *et al.*: **Metanalyses of studies of ventricular enlargement and cortical sulcal prominence in mood disorders. Comparison with controls or patients with schizophrenia.** *Arch Gen Psychiatry* 1995, **52**:735–746.

17. Dupont RM, Jernigan TL, Heindes W, *et al.*: **Magnetic resonance imaging and mood disorders: localisation of white matter and other subcortical abnormalities.** *Arch Gen Psychiatry* 1995, **52**:747–755.

18. Axelson DA, Doraiswamy PM, McDonald WM, *et al.*: **Hypercortisolaemia and hippocampal changes in depression.** *Psychiatry Res* 1993, **47**:163–173.

19. Krishnan KKR, Doraiswmay PM, Lurie SN, *et al.*: **Pituitary size in depression.** *J Clin Endocrinol Metab* 1991, **72**:255–259.

20. Axelson DA, Doraiswamy PM, Boyko OB, *et al.*: **In vivo assessment of pituitary volume with magnetic resonance imaging and systematic stereology: relationship to dexamethasone suppression test results in patients.** *Psychiatry Res* 1992, **44**:63–70.

21. Rubin RT, Phillips JJ, Sadow TF, *et al.*: **Adrenal gland volume in major depression.** *Arch Gen Psychiatry* 1995, **52**:213–218.

22. Goodwin GM, Austin MP, Dougall N, *et al.*: **State dependent changes in brain activity shown by the uptake of ^{99m}Tc-exametazime with single photon emission tomography on major depression before and after depression.** *J Affect Disord* 1993, **29**:243–253.

23. Mayberg HS, Lewis PJ, Regenold W, *et al.*: **Paralimbic hypoperfusion in unipolar depression.** *J Nucl Med* 1994, **35**:929–934.

24. D'haenen HA, Bossuyt A: **Dopamine D_2 receptors in depression measured with SPECT.** *Biol Psychiatry* 1994, **35**:128–132.

25. Mann JJ, Malone KM, Diehl DJ, *et al.*: **Demonstration in vivo of reduced serotonin responsivity in the brain of untreated depressed patients.** *Am J Psychiatry* 1996, **153**:174–182.

26. Schildkraut JJ: **The catecholamine hypothesis of affective disorders: a review of supporting evidence.** *Am J Psychiatry* 1965, **122**:509–522.

27. Coppen A: **The biochemistry of affective disorders.** *Br J Psychiatry* 1967, **113**:1237–1264.

28. Charney DS, Delgado PL: **Current concepts of the role of serotonin function in depression and anxiety.** In *Serotonin Receptor Subtypes: Pharmacological Significance and Clinical Implications.* Edited by Langer SZ, Brunello N, Racagani G, Mendlewicz J. Basel: Karger; 1992:89–104.

29. Potter ZW, Grossman F, Rudoerfer MV: **Noradrenergic function in depressive disorders.** In *Biology of Depressive Disorders, part A: A Systems Perspective.* Edited by Mann JJ, Kupfer DJ. New York: Plenum Press; 1993: 1–27.

Panic and anxiety disorders

Nicholas J. Coupland and David J. Nutt

Normal and pathological anxiety

Fear and anxiety are the emotions normally associated with threatening or aversive situations. Fear refers to immediate threat and anxiety to more distant threats, when these are vague or indeterminate, as in 'free-floating' anxiety, or are expected in the future. They are not uniform states and cognitive, physiological and behavioural dimensions of anxiety have been described, which can vary independently [1]. Neurobiological studies may clarify such relationships by providing a map of the normal processes through which aversive stimuli are evaluated and responses made and of where anxiety disorders deviate from normal. These will probably not show a one-to-one relationship between neurobiological abnormality and diagnostic subgroup. Symptoms and their underlying biology may vary between patients with the same diagnosis; for example, fear, anticipatory anxiety or avoidance could predominate in a phobic person. The boundary from normality may be blurred. Narrowing diagnostic thresholds for public-speaking phobias leads to dramatic drops in prevalence, suggesting a disease continuum, with social determinants, such as occupational roles, cutting across the biology to define cases [2].

Overlapping symptoms are frequent (Fig. 7.1) and patients often have comorbid diagnoses or change diagnosis in time. When symptoms do discriminate, this may be mainly quantitative; for example anxiety attacks in social phobia involve more blushing and difficulty speaking, but less dyspnoea, dizziness and fear of dying than those in panic disorder [3]. The relationship between biological factors underlying predisposition to a disorder and those underlying its expression need to be assessed. For example, post-traumatic stress disorder appears to offer a relatively simple model by virtue of the common aetiological factor of trauma exposure, but premorbid factors, such as childhood abuse and previous psychiatric disorder, also play a role. Factors related to treatment-seeking, including personality, depression and life stresses, may also have biological associations and complicate the interpretation of studies in clinical populations [4].

In this chapter, we will introduce the neurobiology of fear and highlight possible correlates between symptoms and research findings in anxiety disorders, using panic disorder as an illustration. Other approaches may have neurobiological relevance in future; for example, genetic studies have shown higher monozygotic than dizygotic concordance for panic disorder, although heritability was modest. An interesting paradox was that environmental factors were shared in agoraphobic patients but individual for patients with panic disorder [5]. This could support the idea of distinct systems for panic and avoidance but, until relevant genes and their products are isolated, such research remains a step away from neurobiology.

Animal models and human research

Animals cannot model every aspect of human anxiety but studies in animals permit detailed investigation of neurobiological and psychological processes in states in which fear might be inferred, such as responses to acute and repeated aversive stressors. Immediate threats, such as predators or their calls, induce flight, fight or freezing reactions. Conflict tasks involve a behavioural choice, when the animal has learned that action to obtain a reward may also lead to punishment. Tasks that involve novelty also share the potential for risk or reward. Active flight or freezing responses are held in check in these types of task.

Responses may be innate or involve learning processes such as conditioning, sensitization and habituation or extinction. 'Fear conditioning' refers to the development of a conditioned fear response to a previously neutral stimulus after pairing with a fear-inducing aversive stimulus. Conditioning was previously thought to depend purely on the association in time between the stimuli. Modern conditioning theories and experimental evidence support the idea that what the conditioned stimulus predicts about the likelihood or the aversiveness of the unconditioned stimulus is important: experiments that change the pre-

Symptom overlap in anxiety disorders

	Simple phobia	Social phobia	Panic and agoraphobia	Post-traumatic stress disorder	Generalized anxiety disorder
Spontaneous panic			●		
Cued panic or anxiety	●	●	●	●	
Anticipatory worry	●	●	●	●	●
Hyperarousal			●	●	●
Irritability			●	●	●
Avoidance	●	●	●	●	
Derealization and depersonalization			●	●	
Poor concentration			●	●	●
Insomnia				●	●
Nocturnal panic			●		
Nightmares				●	
Flashbacks				●	
Amnesia				●	
Emotional numbing				●	

Fig. 7.1 *Symptom overlap in anxiety disorders.*

dictive value of the conditioned stimulus can change the conditioned response. Such experiments provide the animal with new information about the unconditioned stimulus, which changes its evaluation to being less or more aversive. The conditioned response is then altered without having been directly paired with the newly evaluated aversive stimulus [6].

Innate influences are shown by stronger liability to fear conditioning for 'prepared' or 'prepotent' stimuli, such as spiders or snakes in humans. Fear responses can develop to the environment in which conditioning takes place and this 'contextual conditioning' is most likely after intense aversive stimuli. 'Sensitization' is an increased response on repeated exposure to a stressor and 'cross-sensitization' an increased response when the stressors are different. A decrease in response with repeated stimuli is known as 'habituation' if these are unconditioned and 'extinction' if conditioned. The decrease appears to be due to inhibition rather than a loss of the original response, which can be reinstated rapidly in a different context or after a further stress. 'Active avoidance' has importance in conditioning when the chance exists to escape between the presentation of a neutral stimulus and a paired aversive stimulus. Soon the animal escapes after the first cue and this avoidance delays extinction because the animal fails to learn that the link between the conditioned and aversive stimuli has been broken.

Humans use language and imagery to comprehend and communicate their experiences and the role of these modalities cannot be resolved by animal studies. Nevertheless, the systems controlling fear responses in animals are conserved across evolution into humans and substantial evidence indicates that many of the same conditioning processes are active in humans [6]. The main difference may be that humans can use their capacity for symbolic representations to modify predictions about the unconditioned stimulus. An example would be that individuals informed that their reaction to an electric shock was severe would show a stronger conditioned response than those informed that it was mild, even though no true difference existed.

The interaction between animal and human research is bidirectional and clinical clues help to guide animal studies. For example, various psychological stressors (e.g. life events) and physical stressors (e.g. cocaine abuse, alcohol and benzodiazepine withdrawal) are associated with panic disorder and antidepressants, benzodiazepines and behavioural therapies can be used to treat it. Discovering in animals how these different factors can lead to common endpoints may produce powerful explanatory models. Confirmatory human findings are much harder to obtain. Usually the acquisition phase is long over by the time patients are seen. Until recently peripheral effects of anxiety were far more accessible to study than central ones, for which indirect measures, such as neurotransmitter levels and challenge studies, were needed [7]. Although challenge tests can teach us about anatomically defined systems if a strong background exists in animal studies and the pathways are relatively simple, the interpretation can be very difficult for complex pathways with multiple controls. Human neuroanatomical information was previously only available from lesion and electrode studies in patients with neurological disorders, in whom abnormal limbic discharges during seizure and stimulation are often associated with fear but neuroimaging techniques now becoming available enable central neuronal activity and chemistry to be studied directly.

Neuroanatomical bases of fear and anxiety

Ideas about fear mechanisms can be divided into two concepts. The first is that there is a 'defence system', directed towards making responses to both external threats (e.g. predators) and internal threat (e.g. blood loss, suffocation) and a 'behavioural inhibition' system, involved in suppressing responses that might increase danger. These may operate in concert; for example, in the presence of a predator that is outside attack range, the inhibition system may hold in check both approach and defence reactions that might draw attention. The second concept is that these systems are organized at several levels to meet different processing demands. The amygdala and septohippocampal systems may mediate more automatic processing and exert control over lower areas, such as the hypothalamus or the periaqueductal grey matter, with the 'highest', cortical areas being involved in more cognitively demanding situations (Fig. 7.2).

The amygdala has extensive interconnections with cortex, thalamus, other limbic structures and locus coeruleus, projecting to striatum, midbrain and brainstem to control locomotor, neuroendocrine, autonomic and respiratory responses to threat. Extensive lesioning and neurochemical studies implicate the amygdala in the expression, conditioning and extinction of fear [8]. It is a critical site for kindling, a model process for sensitization, in which subconvulsive electrical stimuli gradually evoke seizures on repetition, until eventually spontaneous seizures occur. Cross-sensitization of defence behaviours may be electrically or chemically induced, for example by gamma-aminobutyric acid (GABA) receptor inverse agonists [9].

Animals must respond to and learn about complex associations of aversive stimuli to allow more discriminating responses than supported by simple conditioning. This requires a comparator system to detect whether the threat or its context is familiar, requiring more automatic responses, or novel, requiring more effort for processing. The hippocampus has been consistently identified as part of a comparator, with different accounts also involving the septum and posterior cingulate and related thalamic nuclei [10]. Different aspects of behavioural inhibition may be mediated by different areas. The medial septum or dorsal hippocampus may be involved in avoidance, so that lesions release approach in conflict tasks. The lateral septum/ventral hippocampus may process safety signals, which are contextual cues indicating decreased danger and allowing approach [11].

The paralimbic cortex (orbitofrontal, insular, anterior temporal, anterior cingulate) links sensory association and premotor and executive areas with the defence and behavioural inhibition systems, mediating emotional influences on more demanding cognitive processing and responses. Patients with paralimbic lesions may show decreases in anxiety, so that lesions to orbitofrontal and cingulate are used as psychosurgical treatments for intractable anxiety disorders. Lesions can also lead to inappropriate emotional responses.

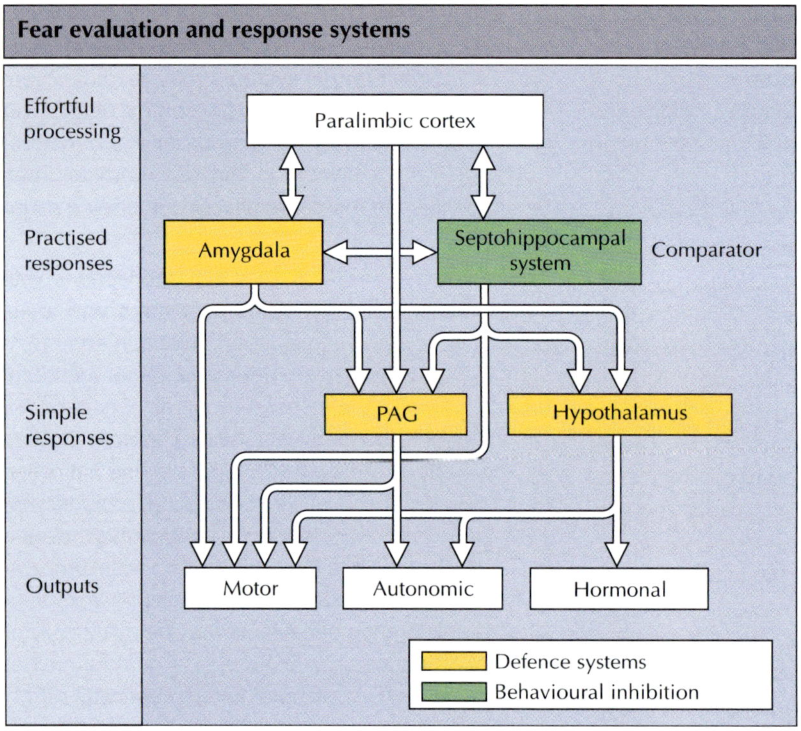

Fig. 7.2 *Fear evaluation and response system. PAG, periaqueductal grey matter.*

The hypothalamus receives widespread limbic and locus coeruleus inputs. It can activate the sympathoadrenal system and releases peptides and releasing hormones, such as corticotropin releasing factor (CRF), vasopressin, oxytocin and growth hormone releasing hormone, in response to aversive stressors.

The periaqueductal grey matter shows topographically organized responses. In addition to descending paralimbic and limbic afferents, ventrolateral periaqueductal grey matter receives deep sensory inputs and stimulation elicits freezing, hypotension, bradycardia and analgesia, adapted to coping with deep injuries. Stimulation in the lateral periaqueductal grey matter produces 'flight' caudally and 'fight' more rostrally. Although both produce tachycardia and increased blood pressure, 'fight' increases facial and 'flight' limb blood flow [12].

Neurotransmitters

Monoamine systems

The monoamine systems consist of nuclei in the midbrain and brainstem, with widespread arborization allowing modulation of many brain areas. The raphe nuclei provide serotonergic innervation to defence, behavioural inhibition and nociceptive systems and autonomic outputs. Electrophysiological studies suggest that raphe projections are mainly influenced by motor activity, firing being quiescent during sleep and increasing through rest to movement [11,13]. The locus coeruleus is the main noradrenergic input to the cortex, limbic areas and thalamus. It is also quiescent in sleep and automatic behaviours, such as grooming, but is activated by novelty, threat and internal stressors, such as hypotension or pain. Noradrenaline release is sensitized by repeated stressors [14,15]. Midbrain dopamine neurones have reciprocal connections with the nucleus accumbens, amygdala and cortex, with prefrontal projections selectively activated by novelty or fear. Other projections that may be recruited by more severe stress are involved in sensitization and cross-sensitization between stress and psychostimulants [16].

How might these systems modulate responses to aversion? Serotonin has been suggested to balance the function of sensory, autonomic and defence systems with the current level of motor activity [11,13]. It inhibits periaqueductal grey matter responses but facilitates higher centres of the defence system. Animals sleep when threats are not expected but must respond quickly to unexpected threat. The periaqueductal grey matter can initiate rapid defence patterns at low levels of arousal, when not restrained by serotonin. During wakefulness, motor activity increases serotonin and shifts control to higher systems, enabling more detailed assessment and controlled responses [13]. Noradrenaline in the cortex suppresses background neuronal activity but facilitates excitatory inputs, improving the precision of sensory inputs. It modifies thalamocortical activity from that of sleep to wakefulness. Modest locus coeruleus activation may enhance attention to and processing of demanding cues but, when activation is high, attention becomes labile and scanning [14]. Dopamine systems are implicated in arousal, attention, working memory, motivation and locomotor responses [16]. High levels of dopaminergic activity produce increasingly stereotyped motor responses. Such noradrenaline and dopamine responses are consistent with the Yerkes-Dodson inverted-U pattern of enhanced performance at modest levels of stress but decreased performance at aversive levels.

Excitatory and inhibitory amino acids

Unlike the diffuse modulatory monoamine systems, excitatory and inhibitory amino acids have more targeted actions in relays and interneurones. GABA is the main inhibitory neurotransmitter and is modulated by various drugs, including benzodiazepines, neurosteroids and alcohol. Benzodiazepine agonists potentiate the anxiolytic effect of GABA, whereas inverse agonists are anxiogenic and antagonists such as flumazenil block both agonists and inverse agonists [17]. Anxiolysis may occur at several sites. Classically, agonists disinhibit responses in conflict tasks but they also inhibit the activity of monoamine systems, which modulate defence and can directly suppress defence reactions mediated by periaqueductal grey matter. Agonists may also interfere with fear conditioning and extinction. In contrast, inverse agonists may elicit defence reactions from the periaqueductal grey matter [18] and may induce behavioural sensitization [9]. Repeated potentiation of GABA may cause tolerance through a shift towards inverse agonist functions, which then emerge during withdrawal. Stress also alters GABA-A functions and the levels of modulatory substances such as neurosteroids.

Neuropeptides

CRF activates the hypothalamic–pituitary–adrenal axis (HPA), with widespread effects which can be characterized as diverting energy use away from growth and reproduction towards energy mobilization. In addition to acting in the HPA axis, CRF has anxiogenic effects in other brain regions: intra-amygdala CRF antagonists block conditioned freezing and the locus coeruleus can be driven by a CRF2 receptor-mediated input. CRF can also facilitate behavioural sensitization. CRF concentrations are elevated in the locus coeruleus during chronic stress, unlike in the hypothalamus, where vasopressin may take over its stimulatory role [19]. Endogenous opioids are also modulated by stressors and cholecystokinin can excite defence reactions at various sites.

Linking animal studies to human anxiety disorders

On the basis of animal studies, speculative links can be drawn between neurobiological systems and clinical and research findings in anxiety disorders. The links for panic disorder are suggested here; readers are referred elsewhere for a detailed consideration of post-traumatic stress disorder [15] and further reviews [20,21].

Clinical features

The signs and symptoms of panic attacks resemble more controlled versions of those elicited from stimulation of the periaqueductal grey matter in humans and animals. The blushing and tachycardia of social anxiety also resembles caudolateral periaqueductal grey matter activation and blood-injury phobia resembles ventrolateral periaqueductal grey matter effects. Panic may be triggered by interoceptive cues. The paradox of panic during sleep and relaxation might be explained by reduced serotonergic inhibition of the PAG during these states. Although agoraphobia and anticipatory anxiety are strongly associated with panic disorder, they are not inevitable, suggesting that they occur at a different level than panic itself. First attacks develop non-randomly, usually away from home, which may relate to the absence of safety signals. Agoraphobia may develop further through contextual conditioning to the situations in which panic occurs. Panic attacks often begin after life stresses and sometimes with abuse of cocaine or alcohol, which may share the capacity for sensitization [22, 23]. Panic disorder occurring with other phobias is usually secondary and perhaps cued anxiety acts as a sensitizing stressor. High arousal and anticipatory anxiety are frequent between panic attacks and patients show heightened attention to cues related to physical threats. These features may reflect excessive engagement of higher defence areas by increased locus coeruleus and CRF drive, although an alternative view is that the locomotor activity associated with hyperarousal is actually compensatory, maintaining inhibitory serotonergic drive to the periaqueductal grey matter. Depersonalization and derealization are frequent in panic disorder; perhaps due to altered sensory processing with high noradrenergic activity e.g. in thalamus.

Treatment response

Antidepressants increase serotonergic output with chronic treatment [24], which might inhibit periaqueductal grey matter responses directly and by facilitation of higher centres. Although the latter effect means that anticipatory anxiety and avoidance might not be reduced directly, in the longer term, the absence of panic would allow extinction [13]. The noradrenergic effects of tricyclic antidepressants and monoamine oxidase inhibitors may also be important, given the evidence for noradrenergic abnormalities in panic disorder. Because these drugs can increase noradrenaline release, their effects seem paradoxical in that the locus coeruleus is thought to be overactive in panic. A possible explanation comes from research into behavioural sensitization, which tends to occur with intermittent stimuli, whereas, with continuous stimuli, tolerance to the effects of a drug may develop. Perhaps panic is associated with intermittent, sensitizing surges of noradrenaline, whereas treatment produces a continuous and desensitizing increase.

Benzodiazepines are often used to treat panic disorder, although, until evidence was produced for the antipanic effects of high-potency drugs such as alprazolam, they were thought to be effective only for the arousal, anticipatory anxiety and avoidance between attacks, rather than for the attacks themselves. Benzodiazepines decrease monoamine release and their effects may depend on a complex interplay of actions at many sites. High-potency drugs might be needed either because of altered GABA function or because their direct inhibitory effects on the periaqueductal grey matter are offset by the fact that they also decrease inhibitory serotonergic input. Inhibition of the locus coeruleus may reduce hyperarousal. Reduced avoidance may depend on suppression of the amygdala. The repeated calming effect of benzodiazepines may be learned as a safety signal, consistent with how they can be effective long before absorption or even while they are still in the patient's pocket. Their main drawback is tolerance and the rebound of panic during withdrawal, which may be due to a change in GABA receptor function.

Unlike benzodiazepines, antidepressants and $5HT_{1A}$ agonists can worsen panic disorder initially. The reasons are unclear but they acutely decrease serotonergic firing, so their net effects on serotonergic transmission in a region depend on how much the terminal or postsynaptic effects outweigh the decreased firing [13,24]. Perhaps the aversive effects in higher centres outweigh the inhibitory effect in the periaqueductal grey matter initially. Other monoaminergic mechanisms for the initial exacerbation effects are possible, such as an increased release of noradrenaline before tolerance has developed.

Cognitive and behavioural treatments, including exposure *in vivo*, interoceptive exposure, cognitive reframing of symptoms and breathing control, are useful in panic disorder. Exposure *in vivo*, like extinction in animals, does not easily generalize to different contexts and avoidance can be rapidly reinstated after a further panic [25]. Conditioning models are less applicable to spontaneous panic and cognitive theories place the primary fault within risk appraisal system, stating that panic is due either to the catastrophic misinterpretation of bodily symptoms [26] or to fear of the consequences of anxiety symptoms [27]. These explanations do not require neurobiological abnormalities because the problem could be the purely faulty evaluation of threat. However, problems exist with pure cognitive theories of panic, such as the occurrence of nocturnal panic and the fact that many patients do not have catastrophic cognitions [21,28].

Anxiety provocation

Psychological challenges and several substances can provoke panic attacks in humans with varying selectivity for patients with panic disorder (Fig. 7.3). Functional imaging studies have shown increased neuronal activity in defence areas during psychological fear provocation [29,30]. Lactate-induced panic was associated with activation of areas of paralimbic cortex and an area that was not clearly distinguishable between superior colliculus and periaqueductal grey matter [31]. Limbic activation and fear induced by procaine is also interesting because of the similarities between this drug and cocaine, which can cause

Fig. 7.3 *Provocation of panic attacks. GABA, gamma-aminobutyric acid; mCCP, metachlorophenylpiperazine hydrochloride; SSRI, selective serotonin reuptake inhibitors. Adapted with permission [21].*

Provocation of panic attacks

Challenge paradigms	Mechanisms
Lactate	? pH changes (?↑pCO_2)
Bicarbonate	? pH changes, ↑pCO_2
Hypercapnia (5 or 35% CO_2)	↑ pCO_2
Hyperventilation	? ↓pCO_2
Hypertonic saline	↑ CRF/↑Noradrenaline
Doxapram	Respiratory stimulation
Caffeine	? ↓ Adenosine, ?↓ Benzodiazepine
Noradrenergic agents:	
yohimbine	↑Noradrenaline
tricyclic antidepressants	↑Noradrenaline, ?↑5HT
isoprenaline, noradrenaline	Peripheral symptoms
Serotonergic agents:	
chlorimipramine, SSRI	?↑ 5HT
mCPP	5HT receptor stimulation
Benzodiazepine-receptor agents:	
FG 7142 (inverse agonist)	↓ Benzodiazepine/GABA
flumazenil (antagonist)	↓ Benzodiazepine/GABA
Cholecystokinin	? Peripheral/brainstem
Hypoglycaemia	? Peripheral symptoms
Cognitive	Catastrophic misinterpretation

panic disorder [22,32]. These studies provide information on the defence system in anxiety studied directly in humans, although spatial and temporal resolution is limited and this type of study does not tell us why the abnormal activation occurred.

Lactate was the first identified panicogen and because it is metabolized to carbon dioxide, a hypothesis was proposed that panic-disorder patients may have an oversensitive suffocation alarm, because carbon dioxide and other panicogens, doxapram and cholecystokinin, produce respiratory stimulation [33]. However, panic also occurs in response to agents with fewer respiratory effects [21] and hyperventilation is often absent in natural panic, so that wider hypotheses may be needed. One proposal is that panicogens act through cognitions [26], but this again appears too specific because the evidence is inconsistent and panic can occur without catastrophic cognitions [28]. Clinical correlates and neuroimaging studies suggest that panic disorder may be associated with widespread changes across the defence and behavioural inhibition systems and we suggest that the final common output of panic may be activated by various pathways.

Within this framework, panicogens could act directly on defence areas, their projection sites in the brainstem or modulatory sites. The periaqueductal grey matter, hypothalamus and locus coeruleus are responsive to interoceptive signals, perhaps explaining not only the effects of respiratory stimuli but also other panicogens, such as hypertonic saline solution, which provokes excitatory CRF drive. Cholecystokinin may directly stimulate brainstem output nuclei, which are relatively unprotected by the blood–brain barrier. Although it excites other areas in the defence system, whether it reaches these after systemic dosage is unclear. Serotonergic drugs may modulate the periaqueductal grey matter or higher centres, although detailed understanding of why some are panicogenic and others not awaits more selective agonists and antagonists [13]. Yohimbine is an alpha-2-antagonist that is panicogenic in panic disorder, post-traumatic stress disorder and cocaine and opiate withdrawal [22]. Opiates inhibit the locus coeruleus, leading to rebound activation on cessation. Cocaine has noradrenergic effects. Because yohimbine blocks alpha-2-autoreceptors, it may reveal locus coeruleus hyperactivity in these conditions by removing inhibition. A weakness in the noradrenergic hypothesis is that yohimbine is not a highly robust panicogen and the alpha-2-agonist clonidine only partly blocks the panicogenic effect of lactate [34]. This is probably because the locus coeruleus is modulatory and its dysfunction only part of a wider range of abnormalities in panic. An alteration in GABA A receptor function towards inverse agonism could also link several findings, including the provocation of panic by the benzodiazepine antagonist flumazenil, decreased diazepam sensitivity in panic disorder and the blockade of the effects of other panicogens by high potency benzodiazepines [17]. Stress might produce such an alteration by changing GABA receptor numbers or subunit composition or by changing the balance of endogenous agonistic and inverse agonistic chemicals, such as neurosteroids.

Non-anxiogenic challenge tests

Non-anxiogenic challenge tests are reviewed in detail elsewhere [34] but attention can be drawn to several points. First, the apparent lack of anxiety after several challenges that provoke physical symptoms seems to argue against interoceptive cues or cognitive misinterpretation being critical in panic. Properly controlled studies, matched for intensity of physical symptoms, are needed of challenge drugs. Second, blunted growth hormone and increased 3-methoxy-4-hydroxy-phenolglycol (MHPG) responses to the alpha-2-adrenoceptor agonist clonidine are consistent with locus coeruleus overactivity in panic disorder to test this fully [34]. We cannot safely assume that alpha-2-adrenoceptor sensitivity is altered, however, because these differences may depend more on basal locus coeruleus hyperactivity. Third, CRF challenges suggest blunting of adrenocorticotropin responses, consistent with CRF overactivity, but circadian studies suggest that HPA axis abnormalities may be present mainly in subgroups of patients [4]. Studying the relationship between HPA axis and noradrenergic dysregulation would be interesting because CRF may influence both.

The future

Although this review is far from exhaustive, we hope that we have made clear that our state of knowledge is primitive and often based on sketchy and sometimes inconsistent evidence, especially when trying to make the links from animal to human studies. Nevertheless, speculation about those links raises fascinating questions and the field is wide open for research to take these further. Although neuroimaging techniques will probably play a major role in human studies, functional studies will need to move from global measures of symptom provocation to a more fine-grained analysis of psychological and neurochemical processes. This might involve testing how psychological or pharmacological manipulation of a symptom modulates neuronal activity. In addition, although no definitive receptor-binding studies have been made to date in anxiety, methods are becoming available both for these and for other measures of interest, such as serotonin turnover and dopamine release. Predictions for human imaging studies are likely to be highly influenced by animal work and by earlier challenge studies. Challenge studies have the advantage over animal studies that they may help to integrate findings from cognitive behavioural research, which have, to some extent, been developed on a separate track, if not indeed in opposition to biological research.

References

1. Lang PJ: **The application of psychophysiological methods to the study of psychotherapy and behaviour modification.** In *Handbook of psychotherapy and behaviour change: an empirical analysis.* Edited by Bergin AE, Garfields SL. New York: Wiley; 1971:75–125.
2. Stein MB, Walker JR, Forde DR: **Public-speaking fears in a community sample.** *Arch Gen Psychiatry* 1996, **53**: 169–174.
3. Walker JR, Stein MB: **Epidemiology.** In *Social phobia.* Edited by Stein MB. Washington DC: American Psychiatric Press; 1995:43–75.
4. Abelson JL, Curtis GC: **Hypothalamic-pituitary-adrenal axis activity in panic disorder.** *Arch Gen Psychiatry* 1996, **53**:323–331.
5. Kendler KS, Neale M, Kessler R, *et al.*: **A population-based twin study of panic disorder in women.** *Psychol Med* 1993, **23**:397–406.
6. Davey GCL: **Classical conditioning and the acquisition of human fears and phobias: a review and synthesis of the literature.** *Adv Behav Res Ther* 1992, **14**: 29–66.
7. Coupland NJ, Glue P, Nutt DJ: **Challenge tests: assessment of the noradrenergic and GABA systems in depression and anxiety disorders.** *Mol Aspects Med* 1992 **13**:221–247.
8. Davis M: **The role of the amygdala in fear and anxiety.** *Ann Rev Neurosci* 1992, **15**:353–375.
9. Adamec RE: **Lasting effects of FG-7142 on anxiety, aggression and limbic physiology in the cat.** *J Psychopharmacol* 1993, **7**:232–248.
10. Gabriel M: **Discriminative avoidance learning: a model system.** In *Neurobiology of cingulate cortex and limbic thalamus: a comprehensive handbook.* Edited by Vogt BA, Gabriel M. Boston: Birkhauser; 1993:478–523.
11. Handley SL: **5-hydroxytryptamine pathways in anxiety and its treatment.** *Pharmac Ther* 1995, **66**:103–148.
12. Bandler R, Shipley MT: **Columnar organisation in the midbrain periaqueductal gray: modules for emotional expression?** *Trends Neurosci* 1994, **17**:379–389.

13. Jacobs BL, Fornal CA: **5HT and motor control: a hypothesis.** *Trends Neurosci* 1993, **16**:346–352.

14. Valentino RJ, Aston-Jones G: **Physiological and anatomical determinants of locus coeruleus discharge.** In *Psychopharmacology: the fourth generation of progress.* Edited by Bloom FE, Kupfer DJ. New York: Raven Press; 1996:373–385.

15. Charney DS, Deutch AY, Krystal JH, *et al.*: **Psychobiologic mechanisms of posttraumatic stress disorder.** *Arch Gen Psychiatry* 1993, **50**:294–305.

16. Le Moal M, Simon H: **Mesocorticolimbic dopaminergic network: functional and regulatory roles.** *Physiol Rev* 1991, **71**:155–234.

17. Malizia AL, Coupland NJ, Nutt DJ: *Benzodiazepine receptor function in anxiety disorders. In GABA-A receptors and anxiety: from neurobiology to treatment.* Edited by Biggio G, Sanna E, Serra M, Costa E. New York: Raven Press; 1995:115–133.

18. Depoortre R, DiScala G, Angst MJ, *et al.*: **Differential pharmacological reactivity of aversion induced by stimulation of the periaqueductal gray or mesencephalic locomotor region.** *Pharm Biochem Behav* 1990, **37**:311–316.

19. Chalmers DT, Lovenburg TW, Grigoriadis DE, *et al.*: **Corticotrophin-releasing factor peptides: from molecular biology to drug design.** *Trends Pharmacol Sci* 1996, **17**:166–172.

20. Gorman JM, Liebowitz MR, Fyer AJ, *et al.*: **A neuroanatomical hypothesis for panic disorder.** *Am J Psychiatry* 1989, **146**:148–161.

21. Nutt D, Lawson C: **Panic attacks: a neurochemical overview of models and mechanisms.** *Br J Psychiat* 1992, **160**:165–178.

22. McDougle CJ, Black JE, Malison RT, *et al.*: **Noradrenergic dysregulation during discontinuation of cocaine use in addicts.** *Arch Gen Psychiatry* 1994, **51**: 713–719.

23. George DT, Nutt DJ, Dwyer BA, *et al.*: **Alcoholism and panic disorder: is the comorbidity more than coincidence?** *Acta Psychiatrica Scandanavica* 1990, **81**:97–107.

24. Blier P, de Montigny C: **Current advances and trends in the treatment of depression.** *Trends Pharmacol Sci* 1994, **15**:220–226.

25. Gelder MG, Marks IM: **Severe agoraphobia: a controlled prospective trial of behaviour therapy.** *Br J Psychiatry* 1966, **112**:309–319.

26. Clark DM: **A cognitive approach to panic.** *Behav Res Ther* 1986, **24**:461–470.

27. McNally RJ: *Panic Disorder: A Critical Analysis.* New York: Guilford; 1994.

28. Coupland NJ, Nutt DJ: **The neurobiology of anxiety and panic.** In *Cholecystokinin and anxiety: from neuron to behavior.* Edited by Bradwejn J, Vasar E. Austin: R.G. Landes Company; 1995:1–32.

29. Malizia AL, Nutt DJ: **Functional neuroimaging studies in human anxiety disorders.** *Acta Neuropsychiatrica* 1995, **7**:S42–S46.

30. Rauch SL, Van Der Kolk, Fisler RE, *et al.*: **A symptom provocation study of posttraumatic stress disorder using positron emission tomography and script-driven imagery.** *Arch Gen Psychiatry* 1996, **53**:380–387.

31. Reiman EM, Raichle ME, Robins E, *et al.*: **Neuroanatomical correlates of a lactate-induced panic attack.** *Arch Gen Psychiatry* 1989, **46**:493–500.

32. Ketter TA, Andreason PJ, George MS, *et al.*: **Anterior paralimbic mediation of procaine-induced emotional and psychosensory experiences.** *Arch Gen Psychiatry* 1996, **53**:59–69.

33. Klein DF: **False suffocation alarms, spontaneous panics, and related conditions.** *Arch Gen Psychiatry* 1993; **50**:306–317.

34. Price LH, Goddard AW, Barr LC, *et al.*: **Pharmacological challenges in anxiety disorders.** In *Psychopharmacology: the fourth generation of progress.* Edited by Bloom FE, Kupfer DJ. New York: Raven Press; 1995: 1311–1324.

Eating disorders

Hanno Pijl and A. Edo Meinders

Introduction

Each year, eating disorders are diagnosed in a growing number of people. These disorders carry important physical and psychological health risks, and both biological and sociocultural factors contribute to their cause. A better understanding of the biological systems regulating nutrient balance and the disturbances that lead to eating disorders may help us to treat and prevent these diseases. This chapter concerns the neurobiological mechanisms of the eating disorders anorexia nervosa and bulimia nervosa and the importance for clinical practice as far as pharmacotherapy is concerned.

Neurobiology of normal eating behaviour

Energy and nutrient balance are regulated by a complex feedback system between body and brain (Fig. 8.1). A variety of metabolic and hormonal afferent signals inform the brain about the current energy status of the body. Nutrients in the blood, including glucose, free fatty acids and amino acids, act as messengers reflecting recent nutrient intake. Circulating hormonal signals, including corticosteroids, insulin and leptin, provide the brain with long-term information concerning the size of the available energy stores. The brain then integrates these afferent sig-

The feedback system between body and brain that regulates energy balance

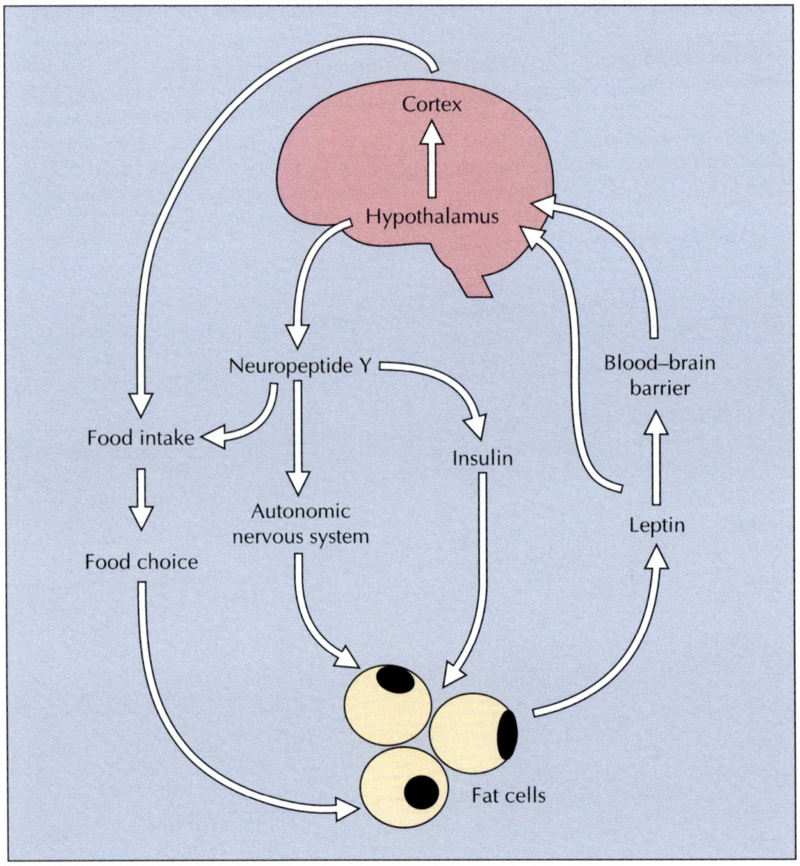

Fig. 8.1 *The feedback system between body and brain that regulates energy balance.*

nals and produces efferent signals that adapt nutrient intake and energy expenditure so that energy balance is maintained.

Several brain areas are involved in the integration of metabolic information. One such area is the hypothalamus, which is closely linked to circulating signals through an extensive vascularity and connection with the pituitary. Several forebrain structures, such as the amygdala and frontal cortex, integrate metabolic information with cognitive factors pertaining to the rewarding or aversive aspects of food.

Many neurochemical systems are believed to modulate the influence of these brain structures on the nutrient intake and energy metabolism.

- Injection of neuropeptide Y into the medial part of the hypothalamus, particularly the paraventricular nucleus, stimulates carbohydrate consumption and reduces energy expenditure.
- Galanin acts within the medial hypothalamus to potentiate fat intake.
- Several other neurotransmitters stimulate food intake and reduce energy expenditure. These anabolic processes are presumably aimed at increasing energy stores (Fig. 8.2).
- The catecholamine dopamine and the tryptophan-derived amine serotonin (5HT) appear to be involved in antagonizing the anabolic signals.
- Dopamine inhibits fat intake and reduces body weight, when injected into the hypothalamus.
- 5HT injection into the paraventricular nucleus reduces food intake, specifically carbohydrate consumption, and probably enhances energy expenditure.

Evidence suggests that disturbances in the endogenous activity of these hormones and neurochemicals are involved in the development of abnormal patterns of eating behaviour and changes in body weight. For example, mice with a phenotype known as ob/ob spontaneously over-eat energy-rich diets and grow obese. These animals are not able to produce leptin, a hormone secreted by adipose cells. When leptin is substituted either by intraperitoneal or intracerebroventricular administration, the ob/ob phenotype reverses and the body weight of the animal returns to that of a normal mouse. This change occurs as a result of a decrease in energy intake and an increase in energy expenditure. Neuropeptide Y appears to be involved in the neurophysiological mechanism that translates the message concerning the size of the adipose tissue stores carried by leptin, into an efferent response. In particular, leptin inhibits neuropeptide Y release in hypothalamic nuclei, thereby inhibiting carbohydrate intake and stimulating energy expenditure. Mice of the phenotype ob/ob characteristically have decreased levels of neuropeptide Y in their brain tissue. Thus, a genetically determined defect in one of the factors that contribute to the regulation of energy balance leads to aberrant eating behaviour and altered body weight. In addition to the genetic predisposition, the presence of specific environmental factors, such as the availability of palatable food, is a prerequisite for the development of the complete phenotype. Evidence suggests that comparable conditions are involved in the pathogenesis of eating disorders in humans.

Anorexia nervosa

Clinical features and epidemiology

A severe disturbance of eating behaviour is a characteristic feature of anorexia nervosa. According to DSM-IV, the diagnostic criteria for anorexia nervosa include refusal to maintain body weight at or above a minimally normal level (85% of what would be expected for age, sex and height), intense fear of gaining weight even when severely underweight, and distorted perception of the shape and size of

Neurotransmitters involved in the regulation of food intake

Inhibiting food intake	Stimulating food intake
Dopamine	Neuropeptide Y
Serotonin	Peptide YY
Corticotropin-releasing hormone	Cortisol
Insulin	Norepinephrine
Cholecystokinin	Galanin
Bombesin	Beta-Endorphin
Somatostatin	

Fig. 8.2 *Neurotransmitters involved in the regulation of food intake.*

the body. In addition, postmenarchal women with anorexia nervosa are amenorrhoeic (Fig. 8.3). Two subtypes of the disease can be distinguished: the 'restricting' type, in which weight loss is primarily achieved by dieting and excessive exercise; and the 'binge eating' or 'purging type', characterized by regular binge eating and purging during the current episode of anorexia nervosa. Personality traits associated with anorexia nervosa differ for the subtypes of anorexics. A restricting anorexic patient is often obsessional, socially inhibited and emotionally restrained. Purging anorexics tend to be more impulsive, emotionally distraught, extrovert and sexually active. Anorexia nervosa is often associated with mood and anxiety disorders, and about half of anorexics have a lifetime history of depression. Social phobia and obsessive–compulsive disorder occur in about 20% of patients. Epidemiological studies indicate that anorexia nervosa is prevalent among adolescent women in Western societies: between 0.5–1% of women in late adolescence and early adulthood meet the full criteria for anorexia nervosa. Only 5–10% of anorexic patients are men, and the disorder is represented equally across the socioeconomic spectrum. The prognosis of anorexia nervosa is poor: only about 40% of patients recover, about 30% improve, while chronic disease develops in 20%. Death occurs in 10% of patients, mainly as a result of electrolyte imbalance, cardiac arrhythmias or suicide.

Pathogenesis

The cause of anorexia nervosa remains unknown. Current theories assume a multifactorial model. Intrinsic biological factors probably determine a trait for developing the disease. Family and twin studies investigating concordance rates provide support for the biological basis of anorexia nervosa. The lifetime risk of acquiring an eating disorder is 2–3 times greater among first degree relatives of patients with anorexia nervosa than among relatives of healthy controls. Furthermore, concordance rates are substantially greater for monozygotic twins than for dizygotic twins. Anorexia nervosa is, however, only found in biologically predisposed persons when other risk factors are present. Sociocultural pressure to be thin (which particularly affects women as a result of gender-role socialization), sexual abuse and certain family interactions have all been recognized as possible risk factors for the development and maintenance of anorexia nervosa. Estimates indicate that genetic factors account for 50–90% of the variance in liability to anorexia nervosa, with the remaining variance explained by environmental factors.

Predisposition to anorexia nervosa

The wide variety of neuroendocrine abnormalities found in anorexic patients are thought to reflect inherited genotypic aberrations. However, almost all endocrine alterations associated with anorexia nervosa, for example hypogonadotropic hypogonadism and increased plasma growth hormone and cortisol levels, can be found in people subjected to dieting or starvation regimens. Moreover, most of the abnormalities are reversed by a return to normal body weight and eating habits. As discussed earlier, food intake and body fat affect brain physiology through a variety of nutritional and hormonal factors that circulate in the bloodstream. Hypothalamo–pituitary function is governed by a wide variety of neurotransmitter systems. Thus, abnormal eating behaviour and low body weight in themselves may cause neuroendocrine changes through their effects on neurotransmitter systems. These changes are, therefore, state-dependent rather than inherited traits. However, some state-dependent endocrine changes, such as hypercortisolism, may perpetuate abnormal behaviour.

DSM-IV criteria for anorexia nervosa

- Refusal to maintain body weight at or above a minimally normal weight for age, sex and height
- Intense fear of gaining weight or becoming fat, even though underweight
- Disturbance in the way in which one's body weight or shape is experienced, undue influence of body weight or shape on self-evaluation, or denial of the seriousness of the current low body weight
- In postmenarchal women, amenorrhea, i.e. the absence of at least three consecutive menstrual cycles

Fig. 8.3 *DSM-IV criteria for anorexia nervosa.*

There are many reasons to hypothesize that a dysregulation of 5HT-mediated neurotransmission is involved in the pathogenesis of anorexia nervosa. First, 5HT in the brain plays a role in the complex mechanisms regulating eating behaviour, and pharmacological enhancement of 5HT neurotransmission in animals and human leads to a reduction in food intake. Second, 5HT is thought to be involved in the pathogenesis of the personality traits and comorbid disorders that are commonly found in patients with anorexia nervosa. 5HT regulates the response of neurobehavioural systems to stimulus events and modulates sexual behaviour and reward motivation for exploring novel environments. Ample evidence suggests that 5HT is involved in the pathogenesis of major depression and obsessive–compulsive disorder. Third, experiments with psychedelic drugs which act via 5HT receptors suggest that 5HT modulates the perception of self and body. Finally, the serotonergic system appears to be more responsive to stimulus perturbations in females than in males, which might explain the gender differences in the risk of developing anorexia nervosa. Neuroendocrine studies consistently reveal reduced 5HT synthesis, uptake and turnover and decreased postsynaptic ($5HT_1$) receptor function in anorexic patients with active disease. All parameters tend to normalize when normal eating patterns return, except for postsynaptic receptor function which remains disturbed until at least 3 weeks after weight restoration [1]. Although decreased central 5HT tone might contribute to the development of several comorbid states and the disturbed body image of anorexia nervosa patients, it is unlikely to be involved in the characteristic inhibition of eating behaviour. Conversely, fasting reduces brain 5HT synthesis and release by diminishing the availability of tryptophan, the precursor amino acid of 5HT. Interestingly, cerebrospinal fluid (CSF) in patients who have recovered and maintained their weight over the long term contains high levels of 5-hydroxy indolic acid (5-HIAA), a major metabolite of brain 5HT. From these data, the following theoretical role of 5HT in the pathogenesis of anorexia nervosa is emerging. Enhanced 5HT turnover and activity might be an inherited trait of patients with anorexia nervosa. High levels of serotonergic activity may shape behavioural propensities toward rigidity and constraint and dampen eating behaviour. These propensities then predispose to the development of anorexia nervosa, which will occur in the presence of other external risk factors. Fasting, in turn, inhibits 5HT-mediated neurotransmission, which causes comorbidity and distorted body image on the one hand and neuroendocrine changes that perpetuate abnormal eating behaviour on the other. Within this framework, it seems important to note that there are some data indicating that anorexic patients of the restrictive type are both clinically and neurochemically distinct from those of the purging type. Future research, which is needed to elaborate the role of 5HT in the pathogenesis of anorexia nervosa, needs to take anorexia nervosa subtyping into account.

Pharmacotherapy

Clearly, treatment of a disease with a multifactorial aetiology requires various therapeutic modalities. Factors other than biological ones indisputably play a role in the perpetuation of pathological behaviour. Therefore, pharmacotherapy can never be the sole therapeutic strategy for anorexia nervosa. The American Psychiatric Association has recently published a set of guidelines for the treatment of eating disorders. Within these guidelines, 'track one' therapeutic issues refer to those related to eating, while 'track two' issues relate to other factors relevant to the patient's recovery, for example depression and anxiety. Although it may seem obvious, it is important to state that any treatment plan for anorexia nervosa must include strategies to normalize eating behaviour. Family therapy, cognitive–behavioural therapy and psychodynamic psychotherapy are non-pharmacological treatment strategies that have all been proven effective in anorexia nervosa, although to only a limited extent. Surprisingly few drugs appear to be effective. Treatment with several tricyclic antidepressants, for example amitriptyline, and antipsychotics, such as pimozide or sulpiride, does not normalize eating behaviour. A few open trials have indicated that selective serotonin reuptake inhibitors (SSRI) might work. This is in keeping with theories assuming low 5HT tone in the brain to be a state-dependent and perpetuating feature of anorexia nervosa. If an enhanced brain 5HT tone indeed proves to be a trait-dependent and initiating feature of the disease, monotherapy with SSRIs obviously cannot cure anorexia nervosa. It seems necessary to test the efficacy of these drugs as an adjunct to behavioural and psychodynamic strategies.

Bulimia nervosa

Clinical features and epidemiology

Bulimia nervosa is characterized by recurrent episodes of binge eating and inappropriate compensatory methods to prevent weight gain. Binges occur at least two times a week for three months. The definition of a 'binge' is the consumption of a very large amount of food within a discrete period of time (e.g. two hours), while the patient experiences a sense of lack of control over the eating behaviour (Fig. 8.4). Although it has been suggested that patients specifically crave for carbohydrate-rich food during a binge, more recent data indicate that binge eating is characterized more by abnormal amounts of calories consumed than by specific cravings. Two subtypes of the disease can be distinguished: the 'purging type', in which the patient regularly engages in self-induced vomiting and the misuse of laxatives, diuretics and/or enemas during the current episode; and the 'non-purging type', which is characterized by fasting or excessive exercise as compensatory measures to prevent weight gain. Note that abnormal bodyweight is not included in the diagnosis: in fact almost all bulimia nervosa patients retain their normal weight, although most patients restrict their food intake between binges. In fact, the clinical pictures of purging type anorexia nervosa and bulimia nervosa are quite similar. Some clinicians consider bulimia nervosa to be a variant of anorexia nervosa, the main distinctive feature being the apparently normal bodyweight of bulimia nervosa patients. Personality traits associated with bulimia nervosa include poor impulse control, 'acting out' behaviour, low frustration tolerance and low self esteem. Major depression and obsessive–compulsive behaviour frequently occur among bulimic patients. Bulimia nervosa appears to be a very common disease among adolescent women. Only about 5–10% of patients are men. Surveys indicate that up to 19% of female students report bulimic symptoms. Using more strict diagnostic criteria, point prevalence of bulimia nervosa in community samples appears to be 1–2 % among young females. Bulimia nervosa is much more difficult to detect than anorexia nervosa. Patients usually try to conceal their symptoms because of feelings of guilt and shame. Prognosis is only slightly better than for anorexia nervosa. About 50% of patients are cured by cognitive–behavioural therapy. In 30% of patients the disease follows a relapsing and remitting course. The remaining 20% of patients develop chronic disease. The mortality rate associated with this disorder bulimia nervosa is uncertain but considerably lower than the mortality rate associated with anorexia nervosa.

Pathogenesis

The aetiology of bulimia nervosa, as of anorexia nervosa, is generally assumed to be multifactorial. The importance of genetic factors is strongly supported by twin studies, which indicate that heritabil-

DSM-IV criteria for bulimia nervosa

- Recurrent episodes of binge eating. An episode of binge eating is characterized by both of the following:
  (1) Eating, in a discrete period of time (e.g. within any 2-h period) an amount of food that is definitely larger than most people would eat during a similar period of time and under similar circumstances;
  (2) A sense of lack of control over eating during the episode (e.g. a feeling that one cannot stop eating or control what or how much one is eating).
- Recurrent inappropriate compensatory behaviour in order to prevent weight gain, such as self-induced vomiting; misuse of laxatives, diuretics, enemas, or other medications; fasting; or excessive exercise.
- The binge eating and inappropriate compensatory behaviours both occur, on average at least twice a week for three months.
- Self-evaluation is unduly influenced by body shape and weight.
- The disturbance does not occur exclusively during episodes of anorexia nervosa.

Fig. 8.4 *DSM-IV criteria for bulimia nervosa.*

ity and environmental influences each account for about 50% of the variance in liability to bulimia nervosa. Sexual abuse and sociocultural and family-related influences have been identified as environmental factors involved in the pathogenesis of bulimia nervosa. The activity of many neuropeptide and amine systems involved in the regulation of eating behaviour have been studied in patients with bulimia nervosa in an attempt to identify the neurobiological mechanism responsible for genetic predisposition. For example, in bulimic women blood levels of cholecystokinin (CCK) and associated sensations of satiety feelings appear to be significantly reduced in response to eating. Furthermore, it has been found that CSF concentrations of peptide YY, a neuropeptide from the same family as neuropeptide Y that stimulates food intake, are elevated in patients with active disease. Both changes presumably promote food consumption. Parallel to changes in anorexia nervosa, plasma levels of cortisol and growth hormone are increased in bulimic patients, while hypogonadotropic hypogonadism occurs in about 50% of patients. It is not known whether these neuroendocrine changes associated with bulimia nervosa are an inherited trait of bulimic patients or are state related. In any case they are likely to play a role in the maintenance of the pathological behaviour.

Data support the existence of a diminished activity of central 5HT-mediated neurotransmission in bulimia nervosa patients. As discussed previously, 5HT is involved in the regulation of a great variety of behavioural and neuroendocrine processes. Decreased central 5HT activity probably stimulates feeding behaviour and is supposed to contribute to the development of anxiety and certain types of depressive disorder. Furthermore, it is conceivable that a defect in central 5HT activity leads to poor impulse control and acting out behaviour, characteristic features of the personality of bulimic patients. Thus, reduced 5HT tone in brain tissue may lead to many of the characteristics and associated comorbidity of bulimia nervosa. CSF levels of 5-HIAA are consistently reduced in ill bulimia nervosa patients. One study even indicates that binge frequency correlates with CSF 5-HIAA concentration. In addition, lower CSF 5-HIAA levels appear to persist in high-binge-frequency bulimics after four weeks of abstinence from binge eating during hospitalization, which supports the hypothesis that low 5HT tone in the brain might be an inherited trait. Neuroendocrine challenge tests provide additional support for reduced central 5HT synthesis and receptor function in bulimia nervosa patients with active disease [2]. Finally, several antidepressants appear to have antibulimic properties. SSRIs were found to be as effective as tricyclic antidepressants in the treatment of bulimia nervosa, which suggests that the antibingeing effect of antidepressive drugs is mediated by enhancement of central serotonergic neurotransmission. It is important to note that the antibingeing effect of tricyclic antidepressants does not depend on the presence of depression or relate to the severity of depressive symptoms. However, some studies have shown that depression and anxiety improve along with eating behaviour during antidepressant treatment, corroborating the hypothesis that 5HT might play a role in the pathogenesis of comorbidity associated with bulimia nervosa. Thus, there is strong evidence to support the existence of a diminished activity of central 5HT-mediated neurotransmission in bulimic patients with active disease. Some data obtained in patients who refrained from bingeing during four weeks suggest that a defect in 5HT turnover might be a trait characteristic.

Bulimic patients typically are anxious and depressed prior to a binge. Some studies suggest that binge eating is subsequently used as a kind of 'self-medication'. Also, bingeing leads to an increase of the plasma tryptophan/large neutral amino acid (Trp/LNAA) ratio. Since tryptophan competes with other large neutral amino acids for transport across the blood brain barrier, an increase of plasma Trp/LNAA enhances availability of Trp to brain tissue, which causes an increment of brain 5HT synthesis and release. An increment of central 5HT-mediated neurotransmission might then improve mood and reduce anxiety. Certain studies show that binge eating indeed reduces anxiety in bulimic patients. However, other studies indicate no change or even deterioration of mood after a binge. Thus, the issue of 'self-medication' by means of binge eating remains a matter of debate.

Pharmacotherapy

Parallel to treatment strategies for anorexia nervosa, bulimic patients need pharmacological treatment as an adjunct to cognitive–behavioural, psychodynamic and/ or family therapy. Guidelines for the treatment of eating disorders published by the American Psychiatric Association bear on bulimia nervosa as well as on anorexia nervosa. Fluoxetine, in a dose of 60 mg per day, remarkably reduces binge–purge frequency and depression and improves several subscale scores on the Eating Disorders Inventory (e.g. body dissatisfaction) in patients with bulimia nervosa. Other selective serotonergic drugs (e.g. fenfluramine, trazodone) appear to be effective too. Thus, SSRIs are the drugs of first choice when pharmacotherapy of bulimia nervosa is necessary.

Conclusions

Anorexia nervosa and bulimia nervosa are eating disorders that occur frequently among young women in Western societies. The aetiology of both disorders is considered to be multifactorial. Inherited physiological abnormalities predispose to the development of aberrant eating behaviour and associated comorbidity. Disease occurs when patients are exposed to environmental influences that trigger abnormal behaviour. Nutrient intake and energy balance are regulated by a complex feedback system connecting body and brain. Defects of various hormones and neurotransmitters that are part of this system have been observed in anorexia nervosa and bulimia nervosa. Most of these defects appear to be state-dependent. Some of these state related abnormalities are likely to play a role in the perpetuation of abnormal behaviour. The nature of the inherited traits predisposing healthy people to develop an eating disorder remains to be elucidated. However, some clues indicate that a dysregulation of 5HT-mediated neurotransmission in the brain might be an inherited trait involved in the pathogenesis of both anorexia nervosa and bulimia nervosa and their associated comorbidity.

References

1. Brewerton TD: **Toward a unified theory of serotonin dysregulation in eating and related disorders.** *Psychoneuroendocrinol* 1995, **20**:561–590.

2. Weltzin TE, Fernstrom MH, Kaye WH: **Serotonin and bulimia nervosa.** *Nutr Rev* 1994, **52**:399–408.

Further reading

Brownell KD, Fairburn CG (eds.): *Eating Disorders and Obesity. A Comprehensive Handbook, edn 1.* London: Guilford Press, 1995.

Edwards KI: **Obesity, anorexia and bulimia.** *Med Clin North Am* 1993, **77**:899–909.

Garner DM: **Pathogenesis of anorexia nervosa.** *Lancet* 1993, **341**:1631–1635.

Pijl H, Meinders AE: **Brain serotonin and food selection: history and current perceptions.** *J Serot Res* 1994, **1**: 21–45.

Woodside DB: **A review of anorexia nervosa and bulimia nervosa.** *Curr Probl Pediatr* 1995, **25**:67–89.

Yager J, Andersen A, Devlin M, *et al.*: **Practice guidelines for eating disorders. American Psychiatric Association.** *Am J Psychiatry* 1993, **150**:207–228.

Obsessive–compulsive and Gilles de la Tourette's disorders

James V. Lucey

Introduction

Obsessive–compulsive disorder (OCD) is a mental health disorder characterized by obsessions and compulsions which are repeated, intrusive and senseless [1]. Obsessions are recurrent thoughts, impulses or images that are intrusive or inappropriate [2]. Attempts to suppress obsessions, with some other action or thought, are unsatisfactory and repetitive. Obsessions are the product of the individual's own mind and patients recognise their origin. Compulsions are repetitive obsessional behaviours that patients are compelled to perform, often in response to an obsession. No realistic connection exists between obsessions and compulsions and, at least initially, patients recognise that these experiences are unreasonable. Crucially, obsessions and compulsions cause marked distress and handicap. Their content is distinct from other axis I disorders (if another is present) and not the product of substance abuse or other general medical disorders [2]. Subcategories may be identified such as: predominantly obsessional (which is closely related to depression), predominantly compulsive (which is not so closely associated with depression and may be more amenable to behavioural therapies), and mixed obsessive–compulsive presentation [3].

The cause of OCD is not known. Freud [4] defined obsessions as psychological defences against unacceptable unconscious impulses. In particular, he developed the concepts of anality and anal sadism which proposed that hostile impulses against parents were controlled by obsessive–compulsive behaviours. More recently some theorists regarded obsessions and compulsions as conditioned responses which functioned to reduce anxiety [5]. The relief brought about by the completion of a compulsive ritual reinforces that ritual. Gradually, because of the usefulness of the behaviour in reducing anxiety, it becomes fixed as a learned pattern of behaviour. In contrast, Schilder [6] proposed that OCD may develop following lesions in foetal life, birth trauma, or following toxic or infectious processes. Few researchers or clinicians now believe in a purely psychological or neurobiological explanation of the disorder. As Freud noted in his description of obsessional neurosis, 'biology is a land of unlimited possibilities ... we cannot guess what answers it will return in a few dozen years ... they may be of a kind which will blow away the whole artificial structure of hypothesis' [4].

Modern biological understandings of OCD arise from clinical observation, therapeutic trials and research studies, in neuroendocrinology and functional imaging and genetics. Since its clinical description, by Westphal [7] in the last century, OCD has been associated with movement disorders and neurological conditions thought to involve dysfunction within subcortical structures such as the basal ganglia [8]. Neurosurgical treatments such as subcaudate tractotomy, although now rarely used, are still effective in resistant cases [9]. OCD patients benefit exclusively from pharmacological treatments which are serotonergically mediated [10]. Traditional noradrenergically mediated antidepressants are ineffective [11,12] and a therapeutic response to serotonergic agents occurs whether or not co-morbid depression is present [13]. Neuroendocrine studies support the existence of serotonergic deficits in OCD [14–16] and, in contrast to most affective or anxiety disorders, the neuroendocrine responses of OCD patients to noradrenergic challenge are normal [17,18]. Functional imaging studies using positron emission tomography (PET) or single photon emission tomography (SPET) have found consistent evidence of brain changes in OCD and Gilles de la Tourette's syndrome (GTS) [19]. Brain activity changes have been shown following treatment, whether pharmacological [20] or behavioural [21], and the relationship between compulsive behaviours, anxiety and brain function is becoming clearer [22]. This chapter describes some recent findings in each of these areas and concludes by suggesting future directions for OCD clinical practice and research.

OCD: neurology, movement disorder and psychosurgery

Idiopathic OCD most commonly develops following head injury [23–25], birth injury [26] or temporal lobe epilepsy [27]. Most OCD patients do not have gross cerebral lesions [27], but discrete lesions of the basal ganglia are associated with obsessive–compulsive phenomena [28–31]. By contrast, more subtle neurological dysfunction (indicated by abnormalities of fine motor coordination, involuntary movements, sensory dysfunction and visuospatial errors) may be common in OCD. Hollander *et al.* [32] studied 41 medication-free OCD patients, finding significantly more soft-signs in OCD patients than in 20 healthy control individuals. Neurological ratings of both OCD patients and control individuals were made in face-to-face or videotaped interviews by a neurologist who was blind to the status of the individual. Similar results were found in a study of 39 OCD patients, 43 healthy controls and 23 non-OCD anxiety disorder patients [33]. Furthermore, OCD patients with high scores on a soft-signs neurological investigation have increased ventricular volumes on computed tomography [34].

Movement disorders with striatal involvement are associated with increased incidence of OCD symptoms [28–31,35,36]. OCD symptoms are more common in post-encephalitic Parkinson's disease and Sydenham's chorea [35,37,38] and the presence of chorea implies basal ganglia involvement. Chapman *et al.* [39] reported eight children who developed obsessive rituals following their infection. In another sample of 23 children with Sydenham's chorea, three children developed substantial obsessional symptoms. Comparison subjects with non-choreiform rheumatic fever did not develop obsessional features [36].

GTS is a related chronic neuropsychiatric disorder with clinical and probable genetic links to OCD [40]. The association between OCD and tics is well established [6,41–43]. GTS onset in childhood is characterized by motor and phonic tics which wax and wane in intensity and nearly 70% of GTS patients have interfering obsessive–compulsive symptoms [40,44]. OCD is prevalent in up to 23% of first-degree relatives of GTS probands [40]. In some OCD studies 6% meet criteria for GTS [44]. Tics are repetitive, involuntary, motor actions. They are not designed to produce or prevent some dreaded situation so that, unlike compulsions, tics are purposeless. Nonetheless, tics are prevalent in up to 38% of OCD patients [44]. In one study of 50 OCD out-patients, GTS was rare (2%) but tics were common [45]. Specific forms of OCD, GTS or tic-spectrum disorder may be genetically related [46].

OCD patients resistant to pharmacological and behavioural treatment may still be treated using surgical techniques. For ethical reasons double-blind trials are difficult to justify, and the number of operations is diminishing. Consequently data on neurosurgical treatment of OCD are uncontrolled and difficult to evaluate. Subcaudate tractotomy using yttrium implants results in 'recovery' in 50–60% of patients [9]. Combining lesions of the subcortical prefrontal connections and the cingulate fasiculi in the 'limbic leucotomy' yields reported 'recovery' rates of 70–88%. Cingulotomy in isolation gives recovery rates of 30% [47]. All these procedures interrupt connections between the subcortex and the inferior prefrontal or the cingulate cortex. Their apparent efficacy suggests specific areas of the brain that may mediate obsessive–compulsive symptoms [19].

OCD psychopharmacology, serotonin and neuroendocrinology

In the 1980s the predominant neurobiological hypothesis of OCD stated that abnormal regulation of brain serotonin (5HT) function contributed at least in part to the development of the disorder [48]. 5HT is an indoleamine neurotransmitter synthesized from tryptophan under the influence of tryptophan hydrolase [49]. From the raphe nucleus of the brainstem, 5HT fibres ascend and descend to influence many areas of the brain, especially neocortex, limbic system, thalamus and hypothalamus. A highly regulated pacemaker pattern of activity is characteristic and, consequently, a broad homeostatic function has been suggested for 5HT systems [50].

The superior efficacy of agents which inhibit re-uptake of 5HT is the clinical basis for theories linking 5HT abnormality and OCD. A number of double-blind studies confirm that clomipramine (CMI), an agent with potent 5HT re-uptake inhibition, is significantly better than placebo at reducing the severity of OCD symptoms [51–53] and benefits are seen in both depressed and non-depressed patients [13, 54]. Newer antidepressant drugs with potent 5HT re-uptake inhibition have also been shown to be effective. Fluvoxamine, fluoxetine and zimelidine have all been beneficial [55–57] and all show potent selective 5HT re-uptake inhibition. In contrast, several well established antidepressants that do not selectively inhibit the re-uptake of 5HT are relatively ineffective in treatment of OCD. Nortriptyline, imipramine and amitriptyline [10–12] are all less potent 5HT re-uptake inhibitors that are ineffective in treat-

Fig. 9.1 *Delta prolactin response (maximum baseline) to 30 mg* D*-fenfluramine in three age-matched groups of men: 10 with DSM IIIR obsessive–compulsive (OCD) disorder, 10 healthy men, and 10 with DSM IIIR major depression.*

Delta prolactin response to D-fenfluramine in three groups of men: OCD, depressed and healthy

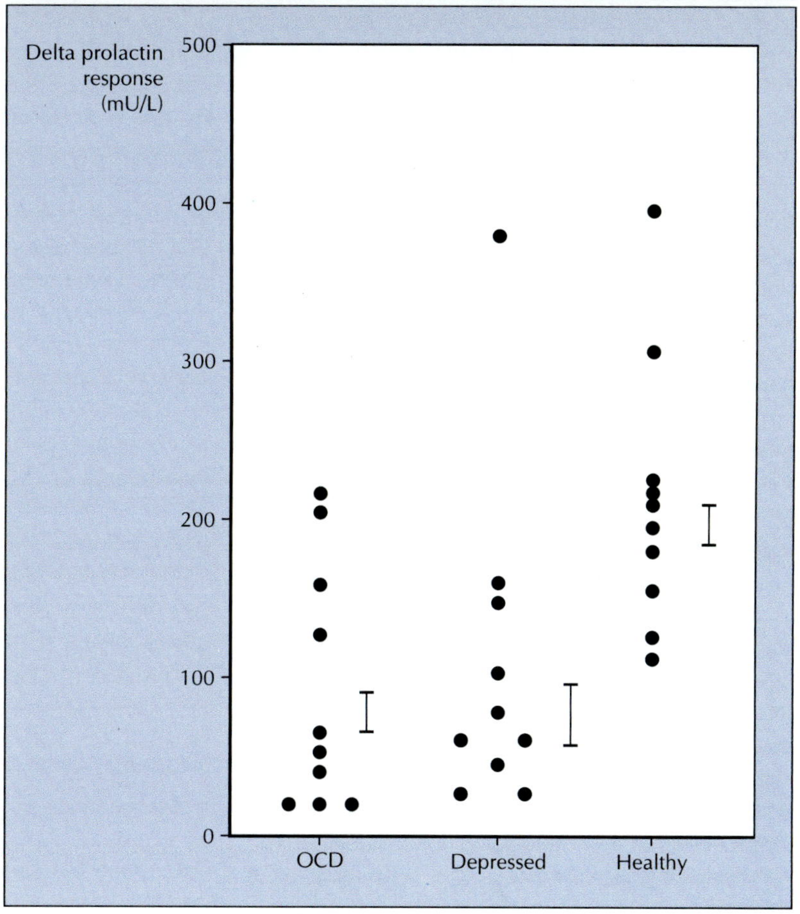

ment of OCD. Leonard *et al.* [58] compared CMI with the potent noradrenaline re-uptake inhibitor desipramine in a 10-week double-blind cross-over trial of 48 children and adolescents with primary OCD. CMI was clearly more effective than desipramine in reducing OCD symptoms. Moreover, 64% of patients who received CMI as their first active treatment showed at least some sign of relapse during desipramine treatment. Goodman *et al.* [59] compared fluvoxamine (a potent 5HT re-uptake inhibitor with no active metabolites) with desipramine and provided further evidence of the specificity of 5HT re-uptake inhibitors in the treatment of OCD.

Neuroendocrine challenge tests allow direct examination of the 5HT system *in vivo [*60]. A rise in plasma levels of pituitary hormones, e.g. prolactin or ACTH, after administrating a serotonergic agent is taken as a measure of the integrity of the hypothalamic–pituitary–serotonergic system. Underactivity or overactivity of the central serotonin pathways is reflected in blunted or enhanced endocrine responses. The D-isomer of fenfluramine releases 5HT from the presynapsis more potently and more specifically than the racemic mixture [61]. 5HT-mediated prolactin and cortisol responses to D-fenfluramine in men with OCD, age matched with depressive men and healthy men, were significantly reduced in OCD compared with healthy controls indicating a deficit of 5HT responsivity in these patients [14] (Fig. 9.1). A similar deficit has been shown in OCD patients responses to 5HT probes mCPP and MK212 [15,16]. However, the reduction in D-fenfluramine-induced 5HT-mediated responsivity in OCD was not distinctive because the responses of patients with major depression were similarly blunted [14]. Although D-fenfluramine response deficits in OCD and in major depression are similar, the extent of neuroendocrine deficit in OCD is much less than in depression. Responses to $5HT_{1A}$ agonism are normal in OCD [62, 63]. The response to the dexamethasone suppression test (a measure of hypothalamic–pituitary–adrenal axis activity) is normal in OCD [64,65]; and (consistent with the failure of noradrenergically mediated antidepressant medication) there is a normal endocrine response to alpha-2 noradrenergic stimulation by clonidine or desipramine in OCD [17,18]. Indirect cholinergic stimulation with the muscarinic agonist pyridostigmine produces a supersensitive growth hormone response in OCD [66], and this is thought to be related functionally to 5HT attenuation, because muscarinic receptors mediating serotonergic inhibition are present on 5HT nerve endings [67]. Thus, compared with affective or anxiety disorders, OCD has a unique neuroendocrine profile: 5HT underactivity and muscarinic supersensitivity in the presence of normal alpha-2 adrenergic activity and normal dexamethasone responsivity [68]. Accordingly, 5HT function is diminished in OCD and its normal tonic inhibitory role may be inadequately performed. Cummings [69] suggests that neuromodulatory substances such as 5HT influence the discharge of dysfunctional cortical–subcortical circuits, such as the inferior frontal/neostriatal circuit. The resultant thalamocortical excitation could contribute to the reverberating pattern of the disorder. This model is useful in integrating neuroendocrine data with neuropsychiatric and neuroimaging findings in the disorder.

OCD functional imaging and the brain

Functional imaging studies using PET or SPET to compare OCD patients with control individuals, have repeatedly found regional differences in OCD cerebral metabolic rates for glucose (rCMG) or OCD cerebral blood flow (rCBF) [70–78]. Despite some variations in results of studies at rest, most report differences in inferior frontal and or medial frontal rCMG; either elevation of OCD rCMG [70–73] or reduction [74,75]. Resting SPET assessment in OCD shows frontal rCBF elevation [76–78] or caudate nuclear (neostriatal) rCBF reduction [22,78,79]. The physiological significance of elevations or reductions is not clear because some state changes could reflect activation and others active inhibition of current mental events. Consequently, whether activity changes (rCBF or rCMG) reflect established features of the disorder (trait) or transient features of symptomatic state should be clarified. Functional imaging using PET adapts well to this study, because repeated scans with low radiation levels can be done within a single session. A PET study of eight OCD patients in resting and provoked (symptomatic) states showed significant increases in rCBF during the activated state in the right caudate, anterior cingulate and bilateral orbitofrontal cortex [80]. In another PET study four OCD males were scanned on 12 successive occasions in the same session, with each scan paired with brief exposure to one of a hierarchy of contaminants that elicited increasingly intense urges to ritualize. OCD patients as a group showed positive correlations between symptom intensity and blood flow to the right inferior frontal gyrus, caudate nucleus, putamen, globus pallidus and thalamus [81]. The data further implicate the orbitofrontal cortex, the cingulate gyrus and the caudate nucleus in the mediating neuroanatomy of OCD [80,81].

Resting OCD SPET studies repeatedly report reduced striatal rCBF [22,78,79] and brain perfusion abnormalities have also been shown in GTS [82]. Fifty GTS patients were compared with 20 healthy controls on rCBF SPET using uptake of 99m-TcHMPAO as a marker of rCBF. Scans were analysed quantitatively using internal ratios to the occipital cortex. GTS patients differed from control individuals in the left caudate nucleus, anterior cingulate, and left dorsolateral prefrontal cortex. Severity of tics was related to hypoperfusion of the left caudate and left medial temporal region [82]. In a similar study of 30 OCD patients compared at rest on 99m-TcHMPAO SPET, rCBF was reduced in seven brain regions including the right inferior frontal cortex, right thalamus and right caudate nucleus (Figs. 9.2–9.4). Two other SPET rCBF studies found similar reduction in caudate rCBF [78,79] and in one study rCBF correlated with increasing anxiety [79]. This apparent paradox could occur as a result of differential responses to separate dimensions of anxiety and OCD. In health, a bell-shaped relationship between anxiety and rCBF is found. The initial linear relationship peaks and further anxiety increases are associated with rCBF reduction [83]. Across studies, OCD groups probably differ, according to state, in their levels of obsessionality and anxiety. Some OCD studies report increased cortical activity (rCBF or rCMG) and others report decreased cortical or subcortical activity. Because variation in

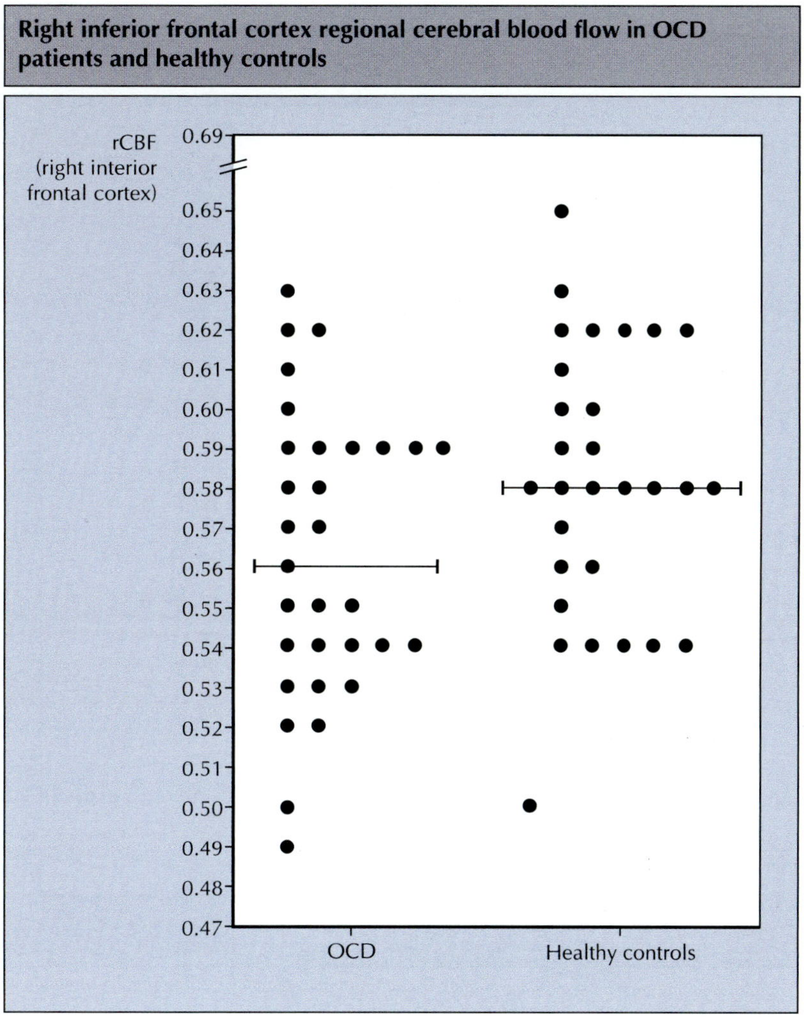

Fig. 9.2 *Right inferior frontal cortical regional cerebral blood flow (rCBF), represented as a ratio of mean cerebellar blood flow in 30 patients with obsessive–compulsive disorder (OCD) and 30 age, sex, and handedness matched control individuals.*

rCBF is related to the mental state [84], differing aspects of OCD and anxiety probably influence separate or even opposing regional rCBF changes [22].

Obsessive–compulsive experience is clinically heterogeneous. A variety of mental mechanisms are probably involved in the mediation of separate features such as recurrent thought, action, anxiety or avoidance. The strength of PET and SPET functional neuroimaging is its ability to relate cerebral activity to these mental processes. Principle component analysis of OCD symptoms in 30 patients who underwent a SPET rCBF scan at rest clearly distinguished obsessive–compulsive from anxious-avoidant symptom dimensions [22]. Obsessive–compulsive correlated negatively with rCBF to the left inferior frontal, medial frontal and right parietal cortex. In contrast, anxious-avoidant correlated positively with rCBF to the right and left caudate, right and left thalami, right inferior frontal, medial frontal and right and left superior frontal cortex. Thus differing clinical dimensions correlated with rCBF in opposing directions, suggesting functional as well as regional distinctions between components of OCD [22].

Recent PET studies have shown that, with successful treatment, changes in cerebral activity occur in OCD patients, regardless of whether that treatment uses serotonergic agents or behavioural psychotherapy [20,21]. The evidence suggests that both forms of treatment influence a common cerebral substrate [19]. This substrate is likely to involve regions connected by thalamocortical loops thought to be dysfunctional in OCD [69]. This conclusion is consistent with animal data suggesting subcortical structures, such as the caudate nucleus, have an impor-

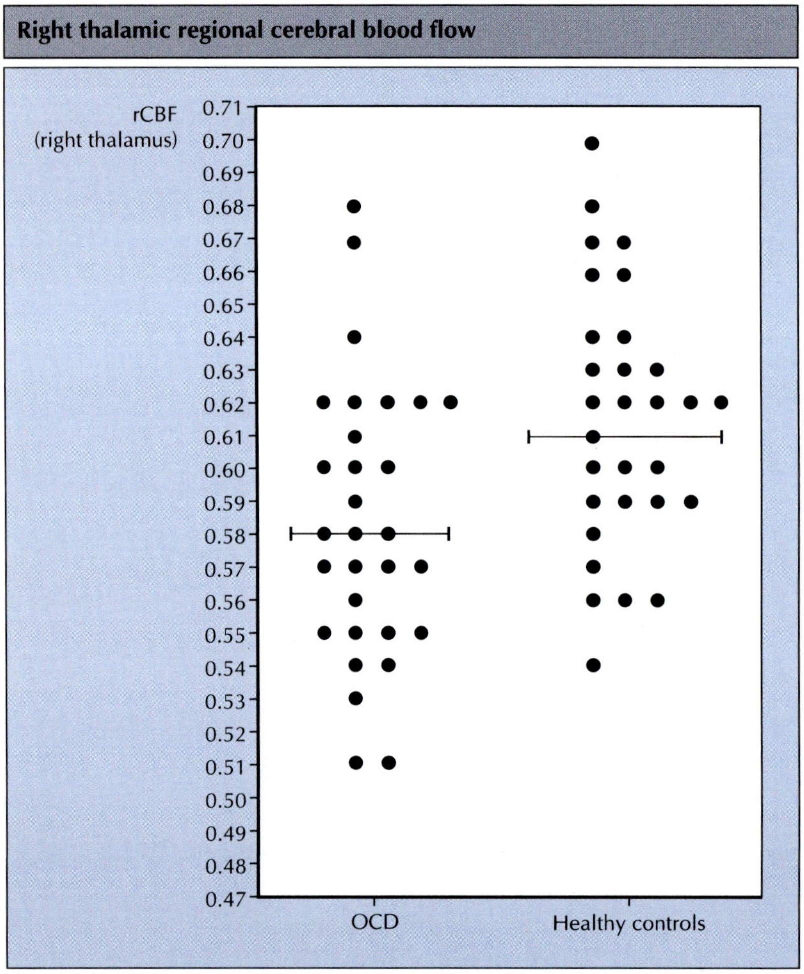

Fig. 9.3 *Right thalamic regional cerebral blood flow (rCBF), represented as a ratio of mean cerebellar blood flow in 30 patients with obsessive–compulsive (OCD) and 30 age, sex, and handedness matched healthy control individuals.*

tant role in higher cerebral function [85] and with other evidence linking OCD to the basal ganglia and their frontal connections [8].

It seems improbable that such consistent functional imaging differences from health could exist in the absence of underlying structural abnormality, however subtle this abnormality might be. Yet to date no consistent picture of structural difference in OCD or GTS has been found. A bilateral reduction in caudate volume was seen on volumetric analysis of CT images [86], but this was not supported by subsequent magnetic resonance (MR) measurements [87, 88]. In fact, one MRI study reported larger right caudate size in patients compared with healthy volunteers [89]. In a recent study by Robinson *et al.* [90] MR images from 26 OCD patients and 26 healthy control individuals were analysed to determine the volumes of various brain structures. The investigators used high-resolution multiple-slice techniques and automated software for measuring volumes of deep brain structures. A significantly reduced caudate nuclear volume was found in OCD patients, but further studies are needed with similarly sophisticated techniques to verify these results.

Genetics

Some twin studies suggest that genetic influences are important in the development of OCD and GTS. Monozygotic concordance rates between 53% and 87% have been reported [91]. Other twin studies suggest genetic factors contribute to the manifestation of anxiety disorders more generally [92]. They argue that genetic data are best interpreted as providing evidence of a general neurotic syndrome [92]. Methodological limitations such as inconsistent diagnostic criteria and lack of comparison groups make

Fig. 9.4 *Right caudate regional cerebral blood flow (rCBF) represented as a ratio of mean cerebellar blood flow in 15 OCD patients, 15 patients with panic disorder with agoraphobia and 15 age, sex and handedness matched control individuals.*

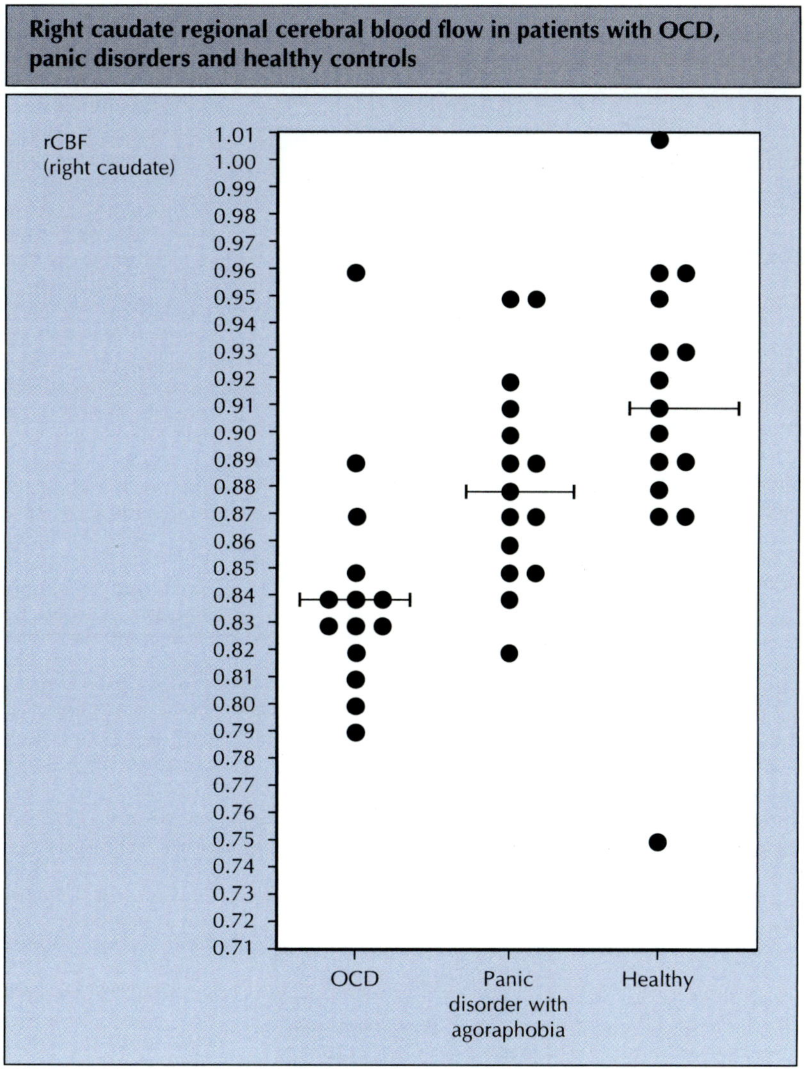

cross-study comparisons difficult. A recent well-conducted family study has helped to redefine the issues [93]. They examined 466 first-degree relatives of 100 probands with obsessive–compulsive disorder and 113 control individuals. Rates of obsessive–compulsive disorder were much higher amongst relatives of OCD probands (10.3%) than the control individuals (2%). The rate of tics (Tourette's syndrome and chronic tics) was significantly higher among the relatives of OCD probands (4.6%) than the control individuals (1%). Relatives of female probands were more likely to have OCD and early onset increased the likelihood of OCD with tics [93]. Once again the authors conclude that OCD is heterogeneous. Some cases are familial and are associated with tics, others are familial and not associated with tics, and a third group has neither family history nor movement disorders.

Conclusion

Over the past decade interest in the biological basis of OCD and GTS has increased. Compelling evidence indicates that OCD is a common, heterogeneous, neuropsychiatric disorder. Long-standing clinical and therapeutic experience contributed to theories that are now supported by biochemical and neuroimaging research data. The potential for molecular biological study of these disorders should soon be realized. Future OCD research must adhere to operational illness definitions, with well defined clinical subgroups. In this way, the relationships between OCD, GTS and CNS dysfunction can be explained.

Acknowledgements

Collection of SPET data in this chapter was supported by a Wellcome Trust Training Fellowship. I wish to acknowledge the support of my colleagues at the Institute of Psychiatry and the Institute of Nuclear Medicine in London.

References

1. Marks IM: *Fears, Phobias and Rituals: Panic anxiety and their disorders*. Oxford: Oxford University Press; 1987: 423–453.

2. American Psychiatric Association: *Diagnostic and Statistical Manual of Mental Disorders, Fourth Edition.* Washington DC: American Psychiatric Association; 1994.

3. World Health Organisation: *The ICD-10 Classification of Mental and Behavioural Disorders: Clinical description and diagnostic guidelines.* Geneva: World Health Organisation; 1992:132–173.

4. Freud S: **Notes on a case of obsessional neurosis.** In *Complete works of Sigmund Freud.* Standard edition 1909, vol 10. London: Hogarth Press; 1955:153.

5. Salzman L, Thaler FH: **Obsessive-compulsive disorder: A review of the literature.** *Am J Psychiatry* 1981, **136**:286–296.

6. Schilder P: **The organic basis of obsessions and compulsions.** *Am J Psychiatry* 1938, **94**:1397.

7. Westphal C: **Dwangforstellungen.** *Arch Psychiatr Nervenkrank* 1878, **8**:734–750.

8. Rapoport JL: **Obsessive–compulsive disorder and basal ganglia dysfunction.** *Psychol Med* 1990, **20**:465–469.

9. Chiocca EA, Martuza RL: **Neurosurgical treatment of the obsessive–compulsive disorder.** In *Obsessive–compulsive disorders: Theory and management.* Edited by Jenike MA, Baer L, Minichiello WE, *et al.* Mosby Year Book, St. Louis. 1990.

10. Thoren P, Asberg M, Cronholm B, *et al.*: **Treatment of obsessive–compulsive disorder with clomipramine, 1: a controlled clinical trial.** *Arch Gen Psychiatry* 1980, **42**: 977–983.

11. Ananth J, Pecknold JC, Van den Steen N, *et al.*: **Double blind comparative study of clomipramine and amitriptyline in obsessive neurosis.** *Prog Neuropsychopharmacol Biol Psychiatry* 1981, **5**:257–262.

12.Volavka J, Neziroglu F, Yaryura-Tobias JA: **Clomipramine and imipramine in obsessive compulsive disorder.** *Psychiatry Res* 1985, **14**:83–91.

13. Mavissakalian M, Turner M, Michelson L, *et al.*: **Tricyclic antidepressants in obsessive–compulsive disorder: anti-obsessional or antidepressant agents?** *Am J Psychiatry* 1985, **42**:572–576.

14. Lucey JV, O'Keane V, Butcher G, *et al.*: **Cortisol and prolactin responses to d-fenfluramine in normothymic obsessive–compulsive disorder, a comparison with depressed and healthy controls.** *Br J Psychiatry* 1992, **161**: 517–521.

15. Bastani B, Nash JF, Meltzer *et al.*: **Prolactin and cortisol responses to MK212 a 5HT agonist in obsessive–compulsive disorder.** *Arch Gen Psychiatry* 1990, **47**:833–839.

16. Hollander E, DeCaria CM, Nitesia A, *et al.*: **Serotonergic function in obsessive-compulsive disorder: behavioural and neuroendocrine responses to m-chlorophenyl piperazine and fenfluramine in patients and normal volunteers.** *Arch Gen Psychiatry* 1992, **49**:21–28.

17. Lee MA, Cameron OG, Guirguis GNM, *et al.*: **Alpha2-adrenoreceptor status in obsessive-compulsive disorder.** *Biol Psychiatry* 1990, **27**:1083–1093.

18. Lucey JV, Barry S, Webb MGT, *et al.*: **The desipramine induced growth hormone response and the DST in obsessive–compulsive disorder.** *Acta Psychiatrica Scand* 1992, **86**:367–370.

19. McGuire PK: **The brain in obsessive–compulsive disorder.** *J Neurol Neurosurg Psychiatry* 1995, **59**:457–459.

20. Benkelfat C, Nordahl TE, Semple WE, *et al.*: **Local cerebral glucose metabolic rates in obsessive–compulsive disorder: patients treated with clomipramine.** *Arch Gen Psychiatry* 1990, **47**:840–848.

21. Baxter L, Schwartz JM, Bergmann KS, *et al.*: **Caudate glucose metabolic changes with both drug and behaviour therapy for obsessive–compulsive disorder.** *Arch Gen Psychiatry* 1992, **49**:690–694.

22. Lucey JV, Costa DC, Blanes T, *et al.*: **Regional cerebral blood flow in patients with obsessive–compulsive disorder at rest: Differential correlates with obsessive–compulsive and anxious avoidant dimensions.** *Br J Psychiatry* 1995, **167**:629–634.

23. Hillbom E: **After effects of brain injuries.** *Acta Psychiatrica Neurologica Scand* 1960, **35(suppl 142)**:125.

24. Lishman WA: **Brain damage in relation to psychiatric disability after head injury.** *Br J Psychiatry* 1968, **114**: 373–410.

25. McKeon J, McGuffin P, Robinson P: **Obsessive compulsive neurosis following head injury — a report of four cases.** *Br J Psychiatry* 1984, **144**:190–192.

26. Capstick N, Seldrup J: Obsessional states: **A study of the relationship between abnormalities occurring at birth and the subsequent development of obsessional symptoms.** *Acta Psychiatrica Scand* 1977, **56**:427–431.

27. Kettl PA, Marks IM: **Neurological factors in obsessive compulsive disorder; Two case reports and a review of the disorder.** *Br J Psychiatry* 1986, **149**:315–319.

28. Laplane D, Baulac M, Widlocher D, *et al.*: **Pure psychic akinesia with bilateral lesions of the basal ganglia.** *J Neurol Neurosurg Psychiatry* 1984, **47**:377–385.

29. Laplane D, Levasseur M, Pilloni B, *et al.*: **Obsessive-compulsive and behavioural changes with bilateral basal ganglia lesions.** *Brain* 1989, **112**:649–725.

30. Denckla MB: **The neurological examination.** In *Obsessive-compulsive disorder in children and adolescents.* Edited by JL Rapoport. Washington DC: American Psychiatric Press; 1989:107–118.

31. Tonkonogy J, Barrieira P: **Obsessive-compulsive disorder and caudate-frontal lesion.** *Neuropsychiatry Neuropsychol Behav Neurol* 1989, **2**:203–209.

32. Hollander E, Schiffman E, Cohen B, *et al.*: **Signs of central nervous system dysfunction in obsessive–compulsive disorder.** *Arch Gen Psychiatry* 1990, **47**:37–32.

33. Bihari K, Pato MT, Hill JI, *et al.*: **Neurological soft-signs in obsessive–compulsive disorder.** *Arch Gen Psychiatry* 1991, **48**:278–279.

34. Stein DJ, Hollander E, Chan S, *et al.*: **Computed tomography and neurological soft signs in obsessive–compulsive disorder.** *Psychiatry Res* 1993, **50**:143–150.

35. Von Economo C: *Encephalitis lethargica: its sequelae and treatment.* London: Oxford University Press; 1931.

36. Swedo SE, Leonard HL: **Childhood movement disorders and obsessive–compulsive disorder.** *J Clin Psychiatry* 1994, **55(suppl 3)**:32–37.

37. Swedo SE, Rapoport JL, Cheslow DL, *et al.*: **High prevalence of obsessive–compulsive symptoms in patients with Sydenham's chorea.** *Am J Psychiatry* 1989, **146**:246–249.

38. Freeman J, Aron A, Collard J, *et al.*: **The emotional correlates of Sydenham's chorea.** *Paediatrics* 1965, **35**: 42–49.

39. Chapman AH, Pilkey L, Gibbons MJ: **A psychosomatic study of eight children with Sydenham's chorea.** *Paediatrics* 1958, **21**:582–595.

40. Pauls DL, Towbin KE, Leckman JF, *et al.*: **Gilles de la Tourette's syndrome and obsessive–compulsive disorder.** *Arch Gen Psychiatry* 1986, **43**:1180–1182.

41. Grimshaw L: **Obsessional disorder and neurological illness.** *J Neurol Neurosurg Psychiatry* 1964, **27**:229–231.

42. Inouye E: **Similar and dissimilar manifestations of obsessive–compulsive neurosis in Monozygotic twins.** *Am J Psychiatry* 1965, **121**:1171–1175.

43. Green RC, Pitman RK: **Tourette's syndrome and obsessive–compulsive disorder.** In *Obsessive–compulsive Disorders: Theory and management.* Edited by Jenike MA, Baer L, Minichiello WE. Littleton: Mass; PSG; 1986.

44. Pitman RK, Green RC, Jenike MA, *et al.*: **Clinical comparison of Tourette's disorder with obsessive–compulsive disorder.** *Am J Psychiatry* 1987, **144**:1166–1171.

45. Lucey JV, Butcher G, Clare AW, *et al.*: **The clinical characteristics of patients with obsessive–compulsive disorder: a descriptive study of an Irish sample.** *Ir J Psychol Med* 1994, **11**:11–14.

46. McDougle CJ, Goodman WK, Price LH: **Dopamine antagonists in tic-related and psychotic spectrum obsessive–compulsive disorder.** *J Clin Psychiatry* 1994, **55(suppl)**:24–31.

47. Jenike MA, Baer L, Ballantine H, *et al.*: **Cingulotomy for refractory obsessive compulsive disorder: a long term follow up of thirty three patients.** *Arch Gen Psychiatry* 1991, **48**:548–555.

48. Insel TR, Mueller EA, Alterman I, *et al.*: **Obsessive–compulsive disorder and serotonin: Is there a connection?** *Biol Psychiatry* 1985, **20**:1174–1188.

49. Aghajanian GK, Sprouse JS, Rasmussen K: **The physiology of the mid-brain serotonin system.** In *Psychopharmacology: The third generation of progress.* Edited by Meltzer HY. New York: Raven Press; 1987:141–150.

50. Steinbush HWM, Mulder AH: **Serotonin-immunoreactive neurones and their projections in the CNS.** In *Handbook of chemical neuroanatomy, classical transmitters and transmitter receptors in the CNS, vol 3, Part II.* Edited by Bjorklund, Hokfelt and Kuhar. New York: Elsevier Science Publishing; 1984.

51. Marks IM, Stern RS, Mawson D, *et al.*: **Clomipramine and exposure for obsessive–compulsive rituals.** *Br J Psychiatry* 1980, **136**:1–25.

52. Flament M, Rapoport J, Berg C, *et al.*: **Clomipramine treatment of childhood obsessive–compulsive disorder.** *Arch Gen Psychiatry* 1985, **44**:219–225.

53. De Veaugh Geiss J, Landau P, Katz R: **Treatment of obsessive–compulsive disorder with clomipramine.** *Psychiatr Ann* 1989, **19**:97–100.

54. Katz RJ, De Veaugh Geiss J, Landau P: **Clomipramine in obsessive–compulsive disorder.** *Biol Psychiatry* 1990, **28**:401–414.

55. Perse TL, Greist FH, Jefferson JW, *et al.*: **Fluvoxamine treatment of obsessive–compulsive disorder.** *Am J Psychiatry* 1987, **144**:1543–1548.

56. Fontaine F, Chouinard G: **An open clinical trial of fluoxetine in obsessive–compulsive disorder.** *J Clinical Psychopharmacol* 1986, **6**:98–101.

57. Prasad AJ: **A double blind study of imipramine versus zimelidine in treatment of obsessive–compulsive neurosis.** *Pharmacopsychiatry* 1984, **17**:61–62.

58. Leonard H, Swedo S, Rapoport Jl *et al.*: **Treatment of childhood obsessive–compulsive disorder with clomipramine and desmethylimipramine. A double blind cross-over comparison.** *Psychopharmacol Bull* 1989, **24**: 93–95.

59. Goodman WK, Price LP, Delgado PL, *et al.*: **Specificity of serotonin re-uptake inhibitors in the treatment of obsessive–compulsive disorder: comparison of fluvoxamine and desipramine.** *Arch Gen Psychiatry* 1990, **47**:577–587.

60. Fineberg N, Montgomery SA: **Neuroendocrine response to serotonergic challenge in obsessive–compulsive disorder.** In *Current Approaches: Obsessive Compulsive Disorder.* Edited by Montgomery SA, Goodman WK, Goeting N. Duphar Medical Publications; 1990:19–25.

61. Garattini S, Mennini T, Samanin R: **From fenfluramine racemate to D-fenfluramine: Specificity and potency of the effects on the serotonergic system and food intake.** *Ann N Y Acad Sci* 1987, **499**:156–166.

62 Lesch KP, Hoh A, Disselkamp-Tietze J, *et al.*: **5-Hydroxytryptamine 1A receptor responsivity in obsessive–compulsive disorder: comparison of patients with controls.** 1991, **48**:540–547.

63. Lucey JV, Butcher G, Clare AW, *et al.*: **Buspirone induced prolactin responses in obsessive–compulsive disorder.** *Int Clin Psychopharmacol* 1992, **7**:45–49.

64. Monteiro W, Marks IM, Noshirvani H, *et al.*: **Normal dexamethasone suppression tests in obsessive–compulsive disorder.** *Br J Psychiatry* 1986, **148**:326–329.

65. Lieberman JA, Kane JM, Sarantokos S, *et al.*: **Dexamethasone suppression tests in patients with obsessive–compulsive disorder.** *Am J Psychiatry* 1985, **142**: 747–751.

66. Lucey JV, Butcher G, Clare AW, *et al.*: **Elevated growth hormone responses to pyridostymine in obsessive–compulsive disorder: evidence of cholinergic supersensitivity.** *Am J Psychiatry* 1993, **150**:961–962.

67. Marchi M, Paudice P, Bella M, *et al.*: **Diclomine and pirenzapine sensitive muscarinic receptors mediate inhibition of ^{3}H-serotonin release in different rat brain areas.** *Eur J Psychiatry* 1986, **129**:353–357.

68. Lucey JV: **Towards a neuroendocrinology of OCD.** *J Psychopharmacol* 1995 **8**:250–257.

69. Cummings JL: **Frontal subcortical circuits and human behaviour.** *Rev Arch Neurol* 1993, **50**:873–880.

70. Baxter LR, Phelps ME, Mazziotta JC, *et al.*: **Local cerebral glucose metabolic rates in obsessive–compulsive disorder.** *Arch Gen Psychiatry* 1987, **44**:211–218.

71. Baxter LR, Schwartz JM, Mazziotta JC, *et al.*: **Cerebral glucose metabolic rates in non depressed obsessive–compulsive disorder.** *Am J Psychiatry* 1988, **145**:1560–1563.

72. Swedo SE, Shapiro MB, Grady CI, *et al.*: **Cerebral glucose metabolism in childhood onset obsessive–compulsive disorder.** *Arch Gen Psychiatry* 1989, **46**:518–523.

73. Nordahl TE, Benkefat C, Semple WE, *et al.*: **Cerebral glucose metabolic rates in obsessive–compulsive disorder.** *Neuropsychpharmacology* 1989, **2**:23–28.

74. Sawle G, Hymas N, Lees A, *et al.*: **Obsessional slowness: functional studies with positron emission tomography.** *Brain* 1991, **114**:2191–2202.

75. Martinot JL, Allilaire JF, Mazoyer BM, *et al.*: **Obsessive compulsive disorder a clinical, neuropsychological and positron emission study.** *Acta Psychiatrica Scand* 1990, **82**:233–242.

76. Zohar J, Insel TR, Berman KF, *et al.*: **Anxiety and cerebral blood flow during behavioral challenge.** *Arch Gen Psychiatry* 1989, **46**:505–510.

77. Machlin SR, Harris GJ, Pearlson GD *et al.*: **Elevated medial frontal cerebral blood flow in obsessive compulsive patients: a SPECT study.** *Am J Psychiatry* 1991, **148**:1240–1242.

78. Rubin R, Villanueva-Meyer J, Ananth J, *et al.*: **Mena I Regional xenon 133 cerebral blood flow and cerebral technetium 99m HMPAO uptake in unmedicated patients with obsessive–compulsive disorder and matched normal controls.** *Arch Gen Psychiatry* 1992, **49**:695–702.

79. Edmonstone Y, Austin MP, Prentice N, *et al.*: **Uptake of 99M-Tc-exametazime shown by single photon emission computerized tomography in obsessive compulsive disorder compared with major depression and normal controls.** *Acta Psychiatrica Scand* 1994, **90**:298–303.

80. Rauch SL, Jenike MA, Alpert NM, *et al.*: **Regional cerebral blood flow measured during symptom provocation in obsessive–compulsive disorder using oxygen 15 labelled carbon dioxide and positron emission tomography.** *Arch Gen Psychiatry* 1994, **51**:62–70.

81. McGuire PK, Bench CJ, Frith CD, *et al.*: **Functional anatomy of obsessive–compulsive phenomena.** *Br J Psychiatry* 1994, **164**:459–468.

82. Moriarty J, Costa DC, Schmitz B, *et al.*: **Brain perfusion abnormalities in Gilles de la Tourettes syndrome.** *Br J Psychiatry* 1995, **167**:249–254.

83. Gur RC, Gur RE, Resnick SM, *et al.*: **The effect of anxiety on cerebral blood flow and metabolism.** *J Cereb Blood Flow Metab* 1987, **7**:173–178.

84 Bench CJ, Friston KJ, Brown RG, *et al.*: **Regional cerebral blood flow in depression measured with positro emission tomography: the relationship with clinical dimensions.** *Psychol Med* 1993, **23**:579–590.

85. Eslinger PJ, Grattan LM: **Frontal lobe and frontal-striatal substrates for different forms of human cognitive flexibility.** *Neuropsychologia* 1993, **31**:17–28.

86 Luxenberg JS, Swedo SE, Flament MF, *et al.*: **Neuroanatomical abnormalities in obsessive–compulsive disorder with quantitative computed x-ray tomography.** *Am J Psychiatry* 1988, **145**:1089–1093.

87 Garber HJ, Ananth JV, Chiu LC, *et al.*: **Nuclear magnetic resonance imaging in obsessive–compulsive disorder.** *Am J Psychiatry* 1989, **146**:1001–1005.

88. Kellner CH, Jolley RR, Holgate RC, *et al.*: **Brain MRI in obsessive–compulsive disorder.** *Psychiatry Res* 1991, **36**:45–49.

89. Scarone S, Colombo C, Livian S, *et al.*: **Increased right caudate nuclear size in obsessive–compulsive disorder.** *Psychiatry Res Neuroimag* 1992, **45**:115–121.

90. Robinson D, Wu H, Munne RA, *et al.*: **Reduced caudate nucleus volume in obsessive–compulsive disorder.** *Arch Gen Psychiatry* 1995, **52**:393–398.

91. Rasmussen SA, Tsuang MT: **Epidemiology and clinical features of obsessive–compulsive disorder.** In *Obsessive compulsive disorders.* Edited by Jenike MA, Baer L, Minichiello WE. Littleton Mass: PSG Publishing Company Inc; 1986:23–44.

92. Andrews G, Stewart G, Allen R, *et al.*: **Evidence for a general neurotic syndrome.** *Br J Psychiatry* 1990, **157**: 6–12.

93. Pauls DL, Alsobrook JP, Goodman W, *et al.*: **A family study of obsessive–compulsive disorder.** *Am J Psychiatry* 1995, **152**:76–84.

Dementia

Michael Kirby and Brian A. Lawlor

Introduction

The term 'dementia' denotes a clinical syndrome with varying causes and pathological features. Many definitions exist but most describe an acquired disorder with global impairment of intellect, memory and personality, occurring in clear consciousness. The concept of global impairment distinguishes a dementia syndrome from focal impairment after a single stroke. However, the cognitive impairment in dementia is rarely truly global and is often characterized by impairment in certain areas of intellectual functioning, with retention of other cognitive functions. The 'acquired' nature of dementia distinguishes it from the cognitive impairment associated with mental handicap. The stipulation of 'clear consciousness' attempts to exclude delirium but may cause diagnostic difficulty in certain situations, such as senile dementia of Lewy body type, which may manifest confusional episodes and have a fluctuating course. Dementia syndromes are usually progressive but not invariably so, such as in some cases of vascular dementia, which may remain stable over time.

In autopsy studies, Alzheimer's disease and vascular dementia are the most frequent causes of dementia, accounting for approximately 48% and 19%, respectively, of all cases, with a further 18% being due to combined Alzheimer's disease and vascular dementia [1–6]. However, these figures may need to be revised downwards on the basis of recent findings that senile dementia of Lewy body type may represent up to 20% of dementia cases in the elderly [7]. Furthermore, some evidence suggests that vascular dementia may occur more often than Alzheimer's disease in people aged more than 85 years [8]. The most frequent causes of dementia are listed in Figure 10.1.

Whereas a definitive diagnosis of the type of dementia requires neuropathological examination, antemortem clinical diagnosis is of more importance to the physician and the identification of reversible or arrestable causes is the primary goal of the diagnostic work-up of patients with a dementia syndrome. Approximately 11% of clinically diagnosed dementia cases are partially or fully reversible, with depression and drugs being responsible for half the cases, followed by metabolic conditions such as thyroid dysfunction and vitamin B12 deficiency, normal-pressure hydrocephalus, subdural haematoma and intracranial neoplasm [9]. As our knowledge of pathogenesis of dementia increases and treatments are developed, the concept of reversible dementia will expand. The routine 'dementia screen' should include a full blood count, serum B12 and folate measurement, biochemical screening, thyroid function tests, syphilis serology, chest radiography, electrocardiography and, ideally, computed tomography (CT) or magnetic resonance imaging (MRI). In patients with an atypical presentation, focal signs or symptoms, myoclonus or where a seizure disorder is being considered, an electroencephalogram may be performed.

The term 'presenile dementia' denotes dementia with age at onset of less than 60–65 years and was initially introduced by Binswanger to distinguish those dementias not dependent on age-related cerebral degeneration. Neuropathological studies have shown little qualitative difference between presenile and senile Alzheimer's disease and the distinction could perhaps be discarded. However, recent molecular genetic work has indicated causative differences between some senile and presenile cases of Alzheimer's disease, lending support to the argument for retention of the distinction.

The more usual categories of dementia will be discussed below, with an emphasis on the recent developments in the underlying biology and the consequent therapeutic implications.

Alzheimer's disease

Alzheimer's disease is the most frequent cause of dementia, representing approximately half of all dementias. In people aged more than 65 years, the prevalence is 5–8%, with an annual incidence of six people in 1000. In most studies, a higher prevalence in women than in men is reported.

Clinical features

Alzheimer's disease manifests with an insidious onset and slowly progressive cognitive impairment. Typical

The most frequent causes of the dementia syndrome

Degenerative
- Alzheimer's disease
- Dementia with Lewy bodies
- Parkinson's disease
- Frontal lobe dementia (Pick's disease)
- Huntington's disease
- Motor neurone disease

Vascular

Toxic
- Alcohol-related dementia
- Drugs*

Infective/Transmissible
- AIDS–dementia complex
- Creutzfeldt-Jakob disease
- Neurosyphilis*

Metabolic and endocrine
- Hypothyroidism*
- Vitamin B12 deficiency*
- Folate deficiency*

Traumatic
- Dementia pugilistica
- Post head injury

Space-occupying lesions
- Chronic subdural haematoma*
- Intracranial neoplasm (primary/metastatic)*

Other
- Normal pressure hydrocephalus*
- Cerebral anoxia
- Depression*

Fig. 10.1 *The most frequent causes of the dementia syndrome. *Potentially reversible causes.*

features in the early stages include the following: impaired learning ability results in poor recall of recent events; expressive language deficits manifest as word-finding difficulties; visuospatial problems may only become obvious in the context of complex tasks such as being unable to orientate oneself in an unfamiliar building or area; mild deficits in abstraction, judgement and calculation may be noted. With progression, memory loss extends to distant events; comprehension becomes impaired; verbal output may degenerate to palilalia and echolalia; agnosia, such as failure to recognise faces (prosopagnosia), and apraxia, such as dressing apraxia, develop; and further deterioration in visuospatial ability, calculation, abstraction, planning and judgement occurs. In contrast with vascular dementia, motor signs and symptoms are absent, except in the late stages, when incontinence and gait abnormalities can develop. The use of standardized criteria for the clinical diagnosis of Alzheimer's disease, such as the National Institute of Neurological and Communicative Disorders and Stroke and the Alzheimer's Disease and Related Disorders Association criteria [10], results in diagnostic accuracy of 80–90%, compared with autopsy [11]; however, the clinical diagnostic accuracy in presenile patients is less. The mean duration of illness for Alzheimer's disease is approximately 10 years but can vary from 2 to 20 years.

Behavioural and psychiatric symptoms (agitation, aggression, wandering, disturbance of sleep and eating patterns, urinary incontinence, delusions, hallucinations, misidentifications and depression) accompany the cognitive deterioration of Alzheimer's disease in up to 75% of patients [12]. Non-cognitive disturbances may develop at any stage of the disease process, impinging greatly on the quality of life of both patient and carer and generally producing greater burden and distress for the carer than the cognitive deficits. Unmodified behavioural disturbances in these patients are a leading cause of hospitalization and institutionalization.

Neuropathology and neurochemistry

Major advances have been made in the understanding of the neuropathology and neurochemical changes of Alzheimer's disease in recent years.

The gross macroscopic changes are non-specific. Total brain weight is reduced with cortical atrophy (which is most marked in the medial temporal regions, especially the parahippocampal gyrus), ventricular dilatation (which is most prominent in the temporal horns of the lateral ventricles) and loss of white matter. Cortical neuronal loss particularly affects large pyramidal cells and is most marked in younger patients. Marked cell loss occurs in the nucleus basalis of Meynert and neuronal loss also occurs in the locus coeruleus and dorsal raphe. The predominant histological features are the presence of neurofibrillary tangles and senile plaques in the hippocampus and cortex. These are seen in other disorders and in normal ageing but their extent and distribution help to identify Alzheimer's disease. The senile plaque is composed of a central core of beta-amyloid protein (bA4), which is derived from the much larger amyloid precursor protein, surrounded by degenerating neurites and located extracellularly primarily in the frontal and medial temporal cortex and the hippocampus. The senile plaque may evolve from a primitive form consisting of bA4 without dystrophic neurites but the presence of these 'diffuse plaques' is not necessarily associated with the presence of dementia. Dystrophic neuronal processes not associated with senile plaques (neuropil threads) are also found in the cortex of patients with Alzheimer's disease and bA4 may be deposited in cerebral arteries, resulting in an angiopathy.

The neurofibrillary tangle is composed of a pair of intertwined filaments (paired helical filaments) and sited intracellularly, predominately in the neurones of the visual and auditory association cortex. The major constituent of the paired helical filaments is an abnormally phosphorylated form of tau, which is a microtubular-associated protein. Alpha-1 antichymotrypsin (AACT), an acute-phase protein, is found within the senile plaques and complement activation occurs in the vicinity of the neurofibrillary tangles and dystrophic neurites, which may implicate abnormal immune-mediated events in the formation of plaques and tangles. The degree of dementia is associated with neurofibrillary tangle count and, to a lesser extent, senile plaque count.

Dysfunction of the cholinergic system is the best described neurochemical deficit in Alzheimer's disease with extensive cell loss in the nucleus basalis of Meynert, which contains the main cholinergic projections to the cortex, hippocampus and amygdala and a reduction in choline acetyl transferase (CAT), the synthetic enzyme for acetylcholine, which has been found to correlate with dementia severity. However, more recently, deficits in multiple neurotransmitter systems, notably the noradrenaline, serotonin, glutamate, dopamine and somatostatin systems, have been described. The clinical correlates of monoaminergic dysfunction are uncertain but may reflect the behavioural and psychiatric complications of Alzheimer's disease [13].

Aetiology

Although the precise cause of Alzheimer's disease remains unknown, genetics and increasing age appear to be the major risk factors. Considerable advances in the genetics of Alzheimer's disease have occurred in the past 10 years. Most cases of Alzheimer's disease are sporadic or apparently sporadic and, although the incidence of Alzheimer's disease increases threefold in first-degree relatives of Alzheimer's disease probands, true autosomal-dominant familial Alzheimer's disease accounts for only 5–10% of all cases and these are predominately of early onset. Much of the molecular genetic work has been concentrated on familial Alzheimer's disease and mutations have been identified at three genetic loci (Fig. 10.2). The interest in the molecular genetics of this small group within Alzheimer's disease arises largely from the information that may be gathered on the functions of the normal gene products and therefore the underlying neurobiology of Alzheimer's disease. Currently, the roles of the normal gene products of APP, presenilin-1 (PS-1) and presenilin-2 (PS-2) remain unclear and proposals for the mechanism by which the gene mutations contribute to the pathogenesis of Alzheimer's disease are speculative but focus on increased production of bA4 and abnormal interactions with cytoskeletal proteins, such as tau.

Apolipoprotein E (apoE) genotype (Fig. 10.2) is the first identified genetic susceptibility factor for the common or so-called 'sporadic' Alzheimer's disease and is also implicated in familial early- and late-onset [17]. ApoE is a polymorphic protein found in many plasma lipoproteins, in which it has a role in lipoprotein metabolism. The apoE gene (APOE) is on the long arm of chromosome 19 and has three common alleles, APOE-ϵ2, APOE-ϵ3 and APOE-ϵ4. The APOE-ϵ4 allele occurs in Alzheimer's disease patients three times more frequently than in normal people. Individuals who are heterozygous for APOE-ϵ4 have a three-fold increased risk of developing late-onset Alzheimer's disease; those who are homozygous have an eight-fold increased risk. However, APOE-ϵ4 alleles are neither necessary nor sufficient for the development of Alzheimer's disease and hence can only be regarded as a susceptibility marker and not a diagnostic marker. APOE genotype also appears to affect the age of onset of Alzheimer's disease with APOE-ϵ4 alleles associated with an earlier onset. The APOE-ϵ2 allele may be associated with a reduced risk for Alzheimer's disease. The function of apoE in the brain and consequently the underlying biological mechanism linking APOE-ϵ4 and Alzheimer's disease are unclear but suggestions include facilitating amyloid deposition and the abnormal phosphorylation of tau proteins.

The lack of 100% concordance for Alzheimer's disease among monozygotic twins and the variability in

Major molecular genetic findings in Alzheimer's disease			
Chromosome		**Gene mutation/allele**	**Affected group**
Autosomal dominant gene mutations			
Amyloid precursor protein [14]	21	4 mutations	5–10% of early-onset FAD
Presenilin-1 [15]	14	28 mutations	70% of early-onset FAD
Presenilin-2 [16]	1	3 mutations	Early and late-onset FAD (Volga-German kindreds)
Susceptibility gene			
Apolipoprotein E gene	19	APOE-ε4	Sporadic and early- and late-onset FAD

Fig. 10.2 *Major genetic findings in Alzheimer's disease. FAD, familial Alzheimer's disease (autosomal dominant).*

age at onset in identical twins suggest that non-genetic factors also play a role. Head trauma and low level of education are the most consistently described putative environmental risk factors for Alzheimer's disease. Head injury might exert its influence through the production of diffuse plaques and low level of education through a reduction in brain synaptic reserve. Genetic and non-genetic factors may interact to increase the risk of Alzheimer's disease, that is a genetic risk may be modified by age, head trauma and other environmental or genetic factors.

Ante-mortem markers

No sensitive or specific ante-mortem marker of Alzheimer's disease currently exists. Structural neuroimaging with CT or MRI is used extensively in the assessment of patients with suspected Alzheimer's disease. CT may show atrophy with sulcal widening and ventriculomegaly but these findings are not diagnostic for Alzheimer's disease and overlap with normal controls is extensive. MRI has greater resolution, is more effective in assessing volume loss and atrophy and can show greater atrophy in the hippocampus and parahippocampal formation in Alzheimer's disease, but again this is non-specific. Functional neuroimaging using single photon emission computed tomography (SPECT) and positron emission tomography (PET) in Alzheimer's disease show tempoparietal deficits on perfusion (SPECT) and metabolism (PET) but lack sensitivity and specificity. The neurochemical abnormalities described above are variable and of little use as ante-mortem markers of Alzheimer's disease. AACT concentrations are elevated in the serum and cerebrospinal fluid of many patients with Alzheimer's disease but this is not specific for the disease. Antibodies to proteins associated with Alzheimer's disease have been developed and proposed as the basis of a possible immunochemical assay for the disease, but their clinical use remains unproven.

Treatment

Most research into treatment strategies for Alzheimer's disease has been concentrated on cognitive symptomatology. The cholinergic deficit has been particularly targeted with the use of acetylcholinesterase inhibitors, such as tetrahydroaminoacridine (THA), which show modest improvement on cognitive measures in at least one-quarter of treated patients [18]. The increase in cognitive scores may be relatively small in responders but can be accompanied by improved quality of life for the patients and should not be underestimated. The major adverse effects of THA are raised serum transaminase concentrations and gastrointestinal disturbances. Markedly raised liver enzyme concentrations occur in almost one-third of patients but are reversible on discontinuation of THA. Currently, THA is approved by the US Food and Drugs Administration and by several other countries. However, neurotransmitter approaches are likely, at best, to provide symptomatic relief for cognitive or behavioural symptoms and are unlikely to alter the underlying disease process.

Inflammatory and immune mechanisms may be involved in the neuropathological process and there is some evidence for a decreased incidence of Alzheimer's disease in patients on long-term drugs with anti-inflammatory properties. It has been suggested that anti-inflammatory or immunosuppressive drugs may have a role in the treatment of the cognitive deficit in Alzheimer's disease. Indomethacin maintained stable cognitive function in a 6-month study [19] but larger trials are necessary. Other therapeutic strategies being investigated include slowing or preventing neuronal death with cytoprotectors such as deferrioxamine and calcium antagonists.

Vascular dementia

The term 'vascular dementia' is preferable to 'multi-infarct dementia' because the underlying disease is not restricted to multiple infarcts and may include ischaemia of the white matter or single infarcts in specific sites. Vascular dementia is recognised as the second most frequent cause of dementia, although some investigators suggest that senile dementia of Lewy body type occurs more frequently than vascular dementia.

Clinical features

Vascular dementia manifests characteristically with an abrupt onset, stepwise progression and fluctuating cognitive impairment. The cognitive deficits tend to be patchy and the clinical picture varies according to the site of the ischaemic lesions, with typical dominant (usually left) hemisphere cortical signs including aphasia, apraxia, agraphia, alexia and acalculia and non-dominant (right) hemisphere lesions producing more marked visuospatial difficulties. If subcortical infarcts predominate, cognitive slowing, dysarthria, incontinence and gait abnormalities may be seen. Focal neurological signs and symptoms and a history of strokes or transient ischaemic attacks may be present. Depressive and psychotic symptoms occur more frequently in vascular dementia than in Alzheimer's disease.

Criteria for the ante-mortem diagnosis of vascular dementia have been proposed by the National Institute of Neurological Disorders and Stroke [20] and by the State of California Alzheimer's Disease Diagnostic and Treatment Center [21]. The Hachinski Ischaemic Score [22] is designed to aid the clinical differential diagnosis of vascular dementia and Alzheimer's disease but has poor inter-rater reliability. Fluctuation in cognitive impairment seen in vascular dementia can cause difficulty in the differential diagnosis from Lewy body dementia.

Neuropathology

In vascular dementia resulting from multiple infarcts, the site of the infarcts may be cortical, subcortical or, more frequently, both cortical and subcortical. A single infarct in certain specific areas of the brain, such as the thalamus or hippocampus, may also produce a dementia syndrome.

White matter ischaemia has been recognised in recent years as an important factor in the pathogenesis of vascular dementia. Binswanger's disease was originally described in 1894 as a rare dementia characterized by loss of white matter and compensatory ventricular enlargement. White matter rarefaction or 'leukoaraiosis', demonstrated by CT or MRI, is now known to occur with much greater frequency than previously assumed, being detected by MRI in almost all patients with vascular dementia and most of those with Alzheimer's disease, although with less severe changes [23]. Up to 38% of normal elderly people have leukoaraiosis detectable on MRI [23] with the incidence increasing with age, and these individuals may have minor cognitive deficits, such as impaired concentration and slowing of mental processing [24]. White-matter lesions are thought to contribute to the pathogenesis of dementia by interfering with subcortical–cortical connections.

Aetiology

Thromboembolic events, usually with a cardiac or carotid origin, are often responsible for the cortical infarcts, although cerebral vasculitis may occasionally be the cause. Deep subcortical infarcts are frequently associated with white matter ischaemia and both tend to occur in hypertensive patients [24].

Investigations

Investigations include routine dementia screening with special attention to potential vascular risk factors. CT or MRI show multiple infarcts or leukoaraiosis, depending on the underlying disease.

Treatment

Evidence indicates that control of vascular risk factors, such as hypertension and smoking [25] and use of an antiplatelet drug can prevent progression in vascular dementia and may even improve cognition. Anticoagulation, in patients with atrial fibrillation, is limited by compliance problems in demented patients. In rare cases, treatment of an underlying vasculitis or hyperviscosity syndrome or surgery for severe carotid stenosis may be indicated. Other specific treatments, such as nootropic agents and calcium antagonists, have been studied but have not been shown to be clinically effective.

Dementia with Lewy bodies

Lewy bodies are filamentous inclusions typically found in the nerve cells of the substantia nigra in Parkinson's disease. Dementia associated with cortical Lewy body formation has aroused considerable interest in recent years and has been variously called Lewy body dementia, diffuse Lewy body disease, senile dementia of Lewy body type and Lewy body variant of Alzheimer's disease. These terms are indicative of the debate whether this dementia syndrome represents a subtype of Alzheimer's disease or belongs to the spectrum of Lewy body disorders (extending from idiopathic Parkinson's disease with predominately subcortical Lewy body distribution to a dementia with subcortical and cortical Lewy body disease).

Clinical features

Clinical and biological features of senile dementia of Lewy body type and Alzheimer's disease are compared in Figure 10.3 [26,27]. McKeith *et al.* [28] found that, using a range of clinical diagnostic criteria, senile dementia of Lewy body type could be misdiagnosed as vascular dementia in up to 35% of patients and as possible Alzheimer's disease in up to 50%. Operational criteria for the clinical diagnosis of senile dementia of Lewy body type have now been developed [29] with good sensitivity and specificity [28].

Neuropathology and neurochemistry

Lewy bodies with neuronal loss occur in the brainstem and subcortical nuclei, including the substantia nigra, locus coeruleus and the basal nucleus of Meynert [29]. Cortical changes include Lewy body formation in the limbic and neocortex and Alzheimer-type disease with numerous senile plaques and few neurofibrillary tangles in most patients, although dementia associated with cortical Lewy body formation has been described without plaques or tangles [30]. Cortical CAT concentrations are markedly reduced and the decreased nigrostriatal dopaminergic activity due to Lewy body disease and neuronal loss in the substantia nigra (Fig. 10.3) may be responsible for the neuroleptic sensitivity seen in patients with senile dementia of Lewy body type.

Aetiology

The cause of senile dementia of Lewy body type is largely unknown, although an increased frequency of the APOE-e4 allele has been found in these patients, similar to that seen with Alzheimer's disease; this may suggest a similarity in disease aetiology between the two disorders [31].

Treatment

The possible greater reduction in CAT concentrations in patients with senile dementia of Lewy body type than in those with Alzheimer's disease (Fig. 10.3) may indicate that the senile dementia of Lewy body type patients will derive greater benefit from anticholinesterase therapies such as THA [32]. The frequent occurrence of psychotic symptoms in senile dementia of Lewy body type may raise the likelihood of neuroleptic medication being prescribed but extreme caution should be exercised in the use of neuroleptics in these patients in view of the increased and sometimes fatal neuroleptic sensitivity which contributes to the reduced survival time compared with Alzheimer's disease [33]. Atypical neuroleptics, with their lower incidence of extrapyramidal side effects, may prove more useful and some favourable reports have been made of the use of respiridone [34].

Dementia in Parkinson's disease

Dementia occurs in approximately 20% of patients with idiopathic Parkinson's disease, although the cause of the dementia syndrome in Parkinson's disease is controversial. Subcortical disease, coexistant Alzheimer's disease and cortical Lewy body formation may be responsible, either alone or in combination. Clinical evidence of subcortical dysfunction (cognitive slowing, attentional deficits, executive function abnormalities) is frequent in Parkinson's disease. Anti-parkinsonian agents may precipitate or aggravate confusion and psychotic symptoms and a balance between the motor disorder and the mental state may need to be achieved.

Frontal-lobe dementia

A degenerative dementia with non-Alzheimer neuropathology affecting the fronto-temporal lobes of the brain with a distinct clinical presentation has been increasingly described in recent years and called variously Frontal-lobe dementia, dementia of frontal-lobe type and non-Alzheimer dementia of frontal-lobe type. Frontal-lobe dementia encompas-

Fig. 10.3 *Comparison of senile dementia of Lewy body type and Alzheimer's disease. APOE, apolipoprotein E gene; CAT, choline acetyltransferase. Variables are compared with age-matched controls as follows: +, mild increase; ++, moderate increase; +++, marked increase; –, mild decrease; – –, moderate decrease; – – –, marked decrease; 0, no change. Adapted with permission [27].*

Comparison of senile dementia of Lewy body type and Alzheimer's disease

	Senile dementia of Lewy body type	Alzheimer's disease
Neuropathology		
Subcortical Lewy bodies	+	0
Cortical Lewy bodies	+++	0
Substantia nigra neurones	– –	0/–
Nucleus basalis of Meynert neurones [26]	– – –	– –
Senile plaques	+++	+++
Neurofibrillary tangles	+	+++
Neurochemistry		
Cortical CAT	– – –	– –
Genetic susceptibility		
APOE allele frequency		
ε2	Normal	– –
ε3	– –	– –
ε4	++	++
Clinical		
Cognitive symptoms	Cortical dementia Insidious onset Fluctuating picture More rapidly progressive	Cortical dementia Insidious onset Minimal fluctuation Slowly progressive
Psychotic symptoms	0/++ (especially visual hallucinations)	0/+
Extrapyramidal symptoms or neuroleptic sensitivity	0/+++	0/+

ses many cases that would have been previously diagnosed as Pick's disease. Some clinicians distinguish between fronto-temporal degeneration with Pick bodies and cells, which they designate Pick's disease, and cases without Pick bodies and cells, which they call frontal-lobe dementia but such a distinction appears to offer little clinical advantage. Frontal-lobe dementia has a predominately presenile age of onset, accounting for 10% of presenile dementias, with an equal incidence between sexes.

Clinical features

The typical manifestation of frontal-lobe dementia is of marked personality change with lack of initiative, lack of concern (which may manifest in a deterioration in personal hygiene or incontinence) and neglect of responsibilities. Affect is shallow with loss of emotional empathy. Some patients are overactive and disinhibited, whereas others may be apathetic, with inertia and lack of spontaneity, and repetitive stereotyped behaviours, such as clapping or singing, may occur. Patients may have changes in sleep and eating patterns. Cognitive deficits are overshadowed by personality and behavioural change but a reduction in the quantity and factual content of speech and difficulties with abstraction, planning and mental flexibility are characteristic, indicating frontal-lobe dysfunction. Memory loss is variable and visuospatial ability relatively preserved. The duration of illness can be 10–15 years and may be longer than Alzheimer's disease.

Neuropathology

Neuronal cell loss, spongiform change and astrocytic gliosis occur in the fronto-temporal cortex and in subcortical structures, with considerable variation in the mix and topographical distribution of these changes. Neurofibrillary tangles, senile plaques and Lewy bodies are absent, and Pick bodies and balloon cells are present in 10–20% of patients [35].

Aetiology

A family history of dementia in a first-degree relative is present in 50% of patients and an autosomal-dominant pattern of inheritance is suggested in studies of extended families with frontal-lobe dementia.

Investigations

The electroencephalogram (EEG) is normal, CT or MRI may show fronto-temporal cerebral atrophy and selective reduction in anterior cerebral blood flow is shown by SPECT.

Frontal-lobe dementia and motor neurone disease

A rapidly progressive frontal-lobe dementia has been described with motor neurone disease [36]. The clinical syndrome of frontal-lobe dementia usually precedes the clinical signs of motor neurone disease. Post-mortem examination shows the neuropathological changes of frontal-lobe dementia with involvement of the fronto-temporal lobes, in addition to degeneraton of the substantia nigra, the hypoglossal nuclei of the brainstem and the anterior horn cells of the spinal cord. Patients usually die after about 3 years as a result of bulbar palsy. Some investigators [37] have proposed that frontal-lobe dementia, motor neurone disease and the combination of the two may represent a clinical range of one pathological spectrum.

AIDS dementia complex

Infection with the human immunodeficiency virus type 1 (HIV-1) may frequently result in disorders of the central nervous system (CNS). A dementing illness directly attributable to HIV-1, rather than an opportunistic infection, is one of the most frequent CNS complications of HIV-1 infection and has been variously named acquired immune deficiency syndrome (AIDS) dementia complex, HIV encephalopathy, HIV dementia and, most recently, HIV-1 associated motor–cognitive complex. AIDS dementia complex is described as a subcortical dementia on the basis of clinical and neuropathological features. Moderate to severe AIDS dementia complex is recognised as an AIDS-defining illness by the US Centers for Disease Control.

Approximately one-third of adults with AIDS may eventually develop AIDS dementia complex [38], although figures of up to 60% have been quoted [39], with moderate or severe dementia occurring in 10–20% . In general, AIDS dementia complex manifests in the later stages of HIV infection when immunosuppression is marked but, in 7% of AIDS patients AIDS dementia complex is among the AIDS-defining illnesses and may be an early manifestation of AIDS [40]. The extremes of age appear to be associated with a higher risk for the development of AIDS dementia complex, with the highest rates in AIDS patients aged less than 15 years or more than 75 years [40]. It is an increasingly frequent cause of dementia in young and middle-aged adults.

Clinical features

Clinically, AIDS dementia complex is characterized by cognitive, motor and behavioural symptoms. Cognitive dysfunction has a subcortical pattern, with mental slowing and concentration and memory difficulties. Motor abnormalities include hand tremor, diminished fine motor control and loss of balance. Behavioural and psychiatric symptoms range from apathy, social withdrawal and irritability to disinhibition, mania and psychotic episodes. The cognitive symptoms and behavioural features such as apathy and lack of interest may result in a diagnosis of depression. In the more severe stages, AIDS dementia complex tends to pursue a rapidly progressive course, although many patients with less severe cognitive impairment show a slowly progressive or even static course.

Neuropathology

Changes predominately occur in the white matter and subcortical gray matter of the basal ganglia and thalamus, with few cortical changes. Reactive astrocytosis, myelin pallor and infiltration by macrocytes, microglia and multinucleated giant cells occur [38]. Earlier reports suggested that neurones were relatively preserved but more recent studies have shown dendritic and synaptic changes and neuronal cell loss [41]. Neuroimaging, especially with MRI, shows generalized loss of white matter and gray matter volume reduction in the basal ganglia and posterior cortex [42].

Pathogenesis

The mechanism by which HIV-1 causes AIDS dementia complex remains speculative. HIV-1 probably enters the brain from both the cerebrospinal fluid and the parenchymal blood vessels [43]. The cells that are directly infected by HIV-1 are the macrophages and microglia but rarely the neurones. Clinical–pathological [44] and clinical–virological [43] studies have shown some discrepancy between histopathological or virological findings and clinical stage, suggesting that direct infection by HIV-1 is not the sole pathogenetic mechanism and that other indirect pathways to tissue injury are involved, which amplify the 'effect of limited brain infection' [43]. HIV infected macrophages, and uninfected macrophages stimulated by HIV-1 proteins may release neurotoxins, such as glutamate-like molecules, free radicals and arachadonic acid, which result in neuronal damage [38].

Treatment

Zidovudine (AZT) has been shown to improve cognitive function in AIDS dementia complex, with PET and SPECT scans showing a corresponding improvement in cerebral function. However, whether this improvement in cognitive function is sustained is unclear because follow-up has been short in most studies. Furthermore, zidovudine may have a neuroprotective role against the development of AIDS dementia complex in cognitively intact AIDS patients, although evidence is conflicting [45]. Patients with AIDS dementia complex may have increased sensitivity to neuroleptic medication, with greater likelihood of developing extrapyramidal symptoms, and caution should be exercised in the use of neuroleptics for the behavioural and psychiatric complications of AIDS dementia complex. The neuroleptic sensitivity may be due to HIV-1 in the basal ganglia with disruption of dopaminergic pathways.

Prion diseases

The prion diseases are a group of relatively rare neurodegenerative disorders afflicting both animals and humans; they are subdivided according to clinical and neuropathological differences. The human prion diseases are Creutzfeldt–Jakob disease (CJD), kuru and Gerstmann–Sträussler–Scheinker disease (GSS); the animal variants include scrapie and bovine spongiform encephalopathy (BSE). The prion diseases have also been known as the 'transmissible spongiform encephalopathies', on the basis of neuropathological findings and the ability to transmit disease by experimental innoculation of animals with infected tissue, and 'slow virus diseases', as a consequence of long incubation periods. However, neither spongiform change nor transmissibilty is universal and no conclusive evidence exists to implicate viruses or viroids. The term 'prion disease' is derived from the accumulation in the brain, probably in neurones, of a pathogenic protease resistant isoform (PrP^{Sc}) of the normal cellular prion protein (PrP^{C}). PrP^{Sc} appears to be the major constituent of the transmissible particle. The precise functional role of the normal prion protein is unclear.

Scrapie, which affects sheep and goats, is the animal prototype of the human prion diseases and the first prion disease to be described. Kuru was described in the early 1950s among the Fore people of New Guinea, in whom it had become an epidemic. The probable origin of kuru in the Fore tribe lay in the sporadic development of the disorder in one person with transmission to others by the ingestion of infected brain as part of ritual cannibalistic practices [46]. Kuru has been virtually eradicated with the cessation of this practice and CJD accounts for the vast majority of human prion diseases. GSS was described in 1936 and is almost always familial, with an autosomal-dominant pattern of inheritance.

The broad clinical features, neuropathology and aetiology of the human prion diseases are outlined in Figure 10.4.

Creutzfeldt–Jakob disease

CJD was first described in the early 1920s, occurs globally, has an incidence of about one per million population, affects both sexes equally and has a peak onset of 60 years.

In more than 85% of patients, CJD appears to be sporadic, with no apparent exposure to the transmissible agent, 5–15% of cases are inherited because of mutations of the PrP gene on chromosome 20, with an autosomal-dominant pattern of disease segregation, and a small number of cases are acquired following infected corneal transplantation, contaminated electroencephalogram electrode implantation or contaminated preparations from human pituitaries such as growth hormone or gonadotrophin. In the case of sporadic disease, either an age-related mutation of the PrP gene occurs, leading to the production of the pathogenic PrP^{Sc}, or PrP^{C} spontaneously converts to PrP^{Sc} in some cells [46]. Molecular genetic studies in 'sporadic' and 'acquired' CJD suggest a possible genetic susceptibility to the development of these disorders in the form of PrP gene variants, specifically homozygosity at PrP codon 129 [47].

Neuroimaging in CJD may be normal or show variable cerebral atrophy and the EEG may show pseudoperiodic sharp complexes.

No specific pharmacotherapeutic treatments exist for CJD or the other prion diseases.

Creutzfeldt-Jakob disease and bovine spongiform encephalopathy

An epidemic of prion disease in cattle (BSE) has occurred in the UK in recent years. The origin of this epidemic is believed to be the practice, banned in 1988, of processing scrapie-contaminated sheep offal into meat and bone meal for cattle feed and, later, also including the rendered carcasses of BSE-infected cows in feed. In 1990, the National CJD Surveillance Unit was set up to monitor changes in the pattern of CJD that might indicate transmission of BSE to humans. The incidence of CJD in the UK has increased in the 1990s but the most likely explanation is improved diagnosis of CJD in the elderly [48]. However, the CJD Surveillance Unit has recently reported 10 patients with CJD, presenting during 1994 and 1995, with a new clinical and neuropathological profile that appears to represent a new variant of CJD and that may be unique to the UK. The unusual features include an earlier age of onset (27 years), a longer mean duration of illness than sporadic CJD (13 months), initial presentation with behavioural and psychiatric symptoms, absence of the typical EEG findings and the consistent neurological finding of PrP plaques that resemble plaques found in kuru and scrapie. Although no direct evidence links this new variant of CJD to exposure to the BSE agent, transmissibility to humans by eating contaminated beef or beef products may be the most plausible interpretation of these findings. The explanation for the young age of the 10 patients remains unclear, with proposed factors being greater exposure through certain foods with high titres of infective material, increased susceptibility to the agent among the young or misdiagnosis of this variant in the elderly [48]. Predictions of the numbers of people who could be affected by this new variant of CJD remains speculative and, if BSE is confirmed as the cause, issues such as the influence of a 'species barrier' that would limit transmission from cattle to humans are unknown. The transmission of scrapie from sheep to humans has never been shown. Animal transmission studies and further epidemiological surveillance are necessary to resolve the issue of a possible link between BSE and CJD conclusively.

Conclusion

Understanding the neurobiology of dementia is of key importance in the development of rational therapeutic interventions for these devastating illness-

Human prion diseases

	Kuru	Creutzfeldt-Jakob disease	Gerstmann-Sträussler Scheinker disease
Age at onset	Variable	Peak at 60 years	20–40 years
Clinical symptoms	Ataxia, tremors, myoclonus & dysarthria	Early rapidly progressive dementia	Chronic cerebellar ataxia
	Progressing to mutism and bulbar involvement	Myoclonus, ataxia, cortical blindness	Slowly progressive
	Dementia (mild)		Possible dementia later
	Death in 1 year	Death in 1 year or less (10% survive >2years)	Death in 5–10 years
Neuropathology	Spongiform degeneration, neuronal loss and gliosis throughout the cerebral grey matter but variable distribution		
Cause	Sporadic initially and subsequently acquired (cannibalism)	85% sporadic, up to 15% inherited, rare acquired cases	Inherited

Fig. 10.4 *Human prion diseases.*

es. Already, in the case of Alzheimer's disease, the demonstration of significant cholinergic deficits has resulted in the use of cholinergic agents and the successful marketing of THA, a cholinesterase inhibitor, for the symptomatic treatment of cognitive impairment in Alzheimer's disease. Improved clinical diagnostic accuracy for vascular dementia allows us to address modifiable risk factors, even in the presence of coexistent Alzheimer's disease and arrest or slow disease progression. The advances in the molecular genetics and biology of Alzheimer's disease and other dementias and the future elucidation of the roles of gene products in the pathogenesis of these illnesses may allow us to modify core neuropathological features and ultimately to provide specific 'gene therapies' for some of the dementias.

References

1. Tomlinson BE, Blessed G, Roth M: **Observations on the brains of demented old people.** *J Neurol Sci* 1970, **11**:205–242.

2. Todorov AB, Go RCP, Constantinidis J, *et al.*: **Specificity of the clinical diagnosis of dementia.** *J Neurol Sci* 1975, **26**:81–98.

3. Molsa PK, Paljarvi L, Rinne JO, *et al.*: **Validity of clinical diagnosis in dementia: a prospective clinicopathological study.** *J Neurol Neurosurg Psychiatry* 1985, **48**:1085–1090.

4. Wade JPH, Mirsen TR, Hachinski VC, *et al.*: **The clinical diagnosis of Alzheimer's disease.** *Arch Neurol* 1987, **44**: 24–29.

5. Jellinger K, Danielczyk W, Fischer P, *et al.*: **Clinicopathological analysis of dementia disorders in the elderly.** *J Neurol Sci* 1990, **95**:239–258.

6. Gilleard CJ, Kellett JM, Coles JA, *et al.*: **The St. George's dementia bed investigation study: a comparison of clinical and pathological diagnosis.** *Acta Psychiatr Scand* 1992, **85**:264–269.

7. Perry RH, Irving D, Blessed G, *et al.*: **Senile dementia of the Lewy body type: a clinically and neuropathologically distinct type of Lewy body dementia in the elderly.** *J Neurol Sci* 1990, **95**:119–139.

8. Skoog I, Nilsson L, Palmertz B, *et al.*: **A population based study of dementia in 85-year-olds.** *N Engl J Med* 1993, **328**:153–158.

9. Clarfield AM: **The reversible dementias: do they reverse?** *Ann Intern Med* 1988, **109**:476–486.

10. McKhann G, Drachman D, Folstein M, *et al.*: **Clinical diagnosis of Alzheimer's disease: report of the NINCDS-ADRDA Work Group under the auspices of Department of Health and Human Services Task Force on Alzheimer's Disease.** *Neurology* 1984, **34**:939–944.

11. Burns A, Luthert P, Levy R, *et al.*: **Accuracy of clinical diagnosis of Alzheimer's disease.** *BMJ* 1990, **301**:1026.

12. Lawlor BA: **Non-cognitive disturbances in Alzheimer's disease.** *Hum Psychopharmacol* 1994, **9**:393–396.

13. Kirby M, Lawlor BA: **Biologic markers and neurochemical correlates of agitation and psychosis in dementia.** *J Geriatr Psychiatr Neurol* 1995, **8**:2–7.

14. Goate A, Chartier-Harlin MC, Mullan M, *et al.*: **Segration of a missense mutation in the amyloid precursor protein gene with familial Alzheimer's disease.** *Nature* 1991, **349**:704–706.

15. Sherrington R, Rogaev EI, Liang Y, *et al.*: **Cloning of a gene bearing missense mutations in early-onset familial Alzheimer's disease.** *Nature* 1995, **375**:754–760.

16. Levy-Lahad E, Wasco W, Poorkaj P, *et al.*: **Candidate gene for the chromosome 1 familial Alzheimer's disease locus.** *Science* 1995, **269**:973–977.

17. Rubinsztein DC: **Apolipoprotein E: a review of its roles in lipoprotein metabolism, neuronal growth and repair and as a risk factor for Alzheimer's disease.** *Psychol Med* 1995, **25**:223–229.

18. Knapp MJ, Knopman DS, Solomon PR, *et al.*: **A 30-week randomized controlled trial of high-dose tacrine in patients with Alzheimer's disease.** *JAMA* 1994, **271**:985–991.

19. Rogers J, Kirby LC, Hempelman SR, *et al.*: **Clinical trial of indomethacin in Alzheimer's disease.** *Neurology* 1993, **43**:1609–1611.

20. Roman GC, Tatemichi TK, Erkinjuntti T, *et al.*: **Vascular dementia: diagnostic criteria for research studies. Report of the NINCDS-AIREN International Workshop.** *Neurology* 1993, **43**:250–260.

21. Chui HC., Victoroff JI, Margolin D, *et al.*: **Criteria for the diagnosis of ischaemic vascular dementia proposed by the State of California Alzheimer's Disease Diagnostic and Treatment Centres.** *Neurology* 1992, **42**:473–480.

22. Hachinski VC, Iliff LD, Zilhka E, *et al.*: **Cerebral blood flow in dementia.** *Arch Neurol* 1975, **32**:632–637.

23. Pantoni L, Garcia JH: **The significance of cerebral white matter abnormalities 100 years after Binswanger's report [Review].** *Stroke* 1995, **26**:1293–1301.

24. Amar K, Wilcock G: **Vascular dementia.** *BMJ* 1996, **312**:227–231.

25. Meyer JS, Judd BW, Tawaklna T, *et al.*: **Improved cognition after control of risk factors for multi-infarct dementia.** *JAMA* 1986, **256**:2203–2209.

26. Forstl H, Burns A, Luthert P, *et al.*: **The Lewy body variant of Alzheimer's disease. Clinical and pathological findings.** *Br J Psychiatry* 1993, **162**:385–392.

27. Harrison RWS, McKeith IG: **Senile dementia of Lewy Body type: a review of clinical and pathological features: implications for treatment.** *Int J Geriatr Psychiatry* 1995, **10**:919–926.

28. McKeith IG, Fairbairn AF, Perry RH, *et al.*: **The clinical diagnosis and misdiagnosis of senile dementia of Lewy body type (SDLT).** *Br J Psychiatry* 1994, **165**:324–332.

29. McKeith IG, Perry RH, Fairbairn AF, *et al.*: **Operational criteria for senile dementia of Lewy body type (SDLT).** *Psychol Med* 1992, **22**:911–922.

30. Gibb WRG, Luthert PJ, Janota I, *et al.*: **Cortical Lewy body dementia: clinical features and classification.** *J Neurol Neurosurg Psychiatry* 1989, **52**:185–192.

31. St Clair D, Norrman J, Perry R, *et al.*: **Apolipoprotein E episilon 4 allele frequency in patients with Lewy body dementia, Alzheimer's disease and age-matched controls.** *Neurosci Let* 1994, **176**:45–46.

32. Wilcock GK, Scott MI: **Tacrine for senile dementia of Alzheimer's or Lewy body type.** *Lancet* 1994, **344**:544.

33. McKeith I, Fairbairn A, Perry R, *et al.*: **Neuroleptic sensitivity in patients with senile dementia of Lewy body type.** *BMJ* 1992, **305**:673–678.

34. Lee H, Cooney JM, Lawlor BA: **The use of respiridone, an atypical neuroleptic, in Lewy body disease.** *Inter J Geriatr Psychiatry* 1994, **9**:415–417.

35. Mann DMA, South PW, Snowden JS, *et al.*: **Dementia of frontal lobe type: neuropathology and immunochemistry.** *J Neurol Neurosurg Psychiatry* 1993, **56**:605–615.

36. Neary D, Snowden JS, Mann DMA, *et al.*: **Frontal lobe dementia and motor neuron disease.** *J Neurol Neurosurg Psychiatry* 1990, **53**:23–32.

37. Talbot PR, Goulding PJ, Lloyd JJ, *et al.*: **Inter-relation between 'classic' motor neuron disease and frontotemporal dementia: neuropsychological and single photon emission computed tomography study.** *J Neurol Neurosurg Psychiatry* 1995, **58**:541–547.

38. Lipton SA, Gendelman HE: **Seminars in medicine of the Beth Israel Hospital, Boston. Dementia associated with the Acquired Immunodeficiency Syndrome.** *N Engl J Med* 1995, **332**:934–940.

39. Navia BA, Jordan BD, Price RW: **The AIDS dementia complex: I. Clinical features.** *Ann Neurol* 1986, **19**:517–524.

40. Janssen RS, Nwanyanwu OC, Selik RM, *et al.*: **Epidemiology of human immunodeficiency virus encephalopathy in the United States.** *Neurology* 1992, **42**:1472–1476.

41. Wiley CA, Masliah E, Morey M, *et al.*: **Neocortical damage during HIV infection.** *Ann Neurol* 1991, **29**:651–657.

42. Aylward EH, Brettschneider PD, McArthur JC, *et al.*: **Magnetic resonance imaging measurement of gray matter volume reductions in HIV dementia.** *Am J Psychiatry* 1995, **152**:987–994.

43. Brew BJ, Rosenblum M, Cronin K, *et al.*: **AIDS dementia complex and HIV-1 brain infection: clinical-virological correlations.** *Ann Neurol* 1995, **38**:563–570.

44. Glass JD, Wesselingh SL, Selnes OA, *et al.*: **Clinical-neuropathologic correlation in HIV-associated dementia.** *Neurology* 1993, **43**:2230–2237.

45. Portegies P: **Review of antiretroviral therapy in the prevention of HIV-related AIDS dementia complex (ADC).** *Drugs* 1995, **49**:25–31.

46. DeArmond SJ, Prusiner SB: **Etiology and pathogenesis of prion diseases.** *Am J Pathol* 1991, **146**:785–811.

47. Palmer MS, Dryden AJ, Hughes JT, *et al.*: **Homozygous prion protein genotype predisposes to sporadic Creutzfeldt-Jakob disease.** *Nature* 1991, **352**:340–342.

48. Will RG, Ironside JW, Zeidler M, *et al.*: **A new variant of Creutzfeldt-Jakob disease in the UK.** *Lancet* 1996, **347**:921–925.

Index